THE FEARLESS FLYER

How to Fly in Comfort and without Trepidation

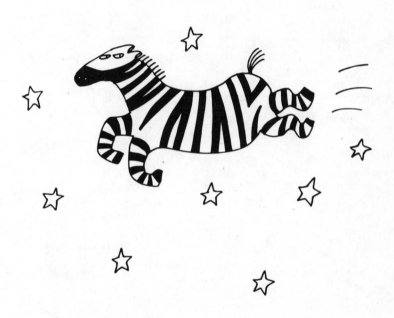

The Fearless Flyer

HOW *to* FLY *in* COMFORT *and* WITHOUT TREPIDATION

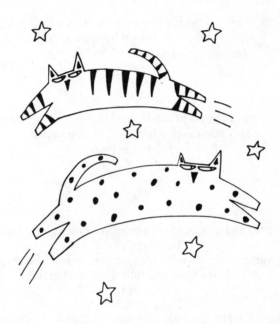

CHERRY HARTMAN
JULIE SHELDON HUFFAKER

Illustrations by Nancy Coffelt

The Eighth Mountain Press
Portland, Oregon · 1995

Cover art and illustrations by Nancy Coffelt
Cover and book design by Ruth Gundle
Technical assistance by Thad Laughlin

Manufactured in the United States of America
This book is printed on acid-free paper.
First edition 1995
10 9 8 7 6 5 4 3 2 1

LIBRARY OF CONGRESS CATALOGING-IN-PUBLICATION DATA
Hartman, Cherry.
The fearless flyer : how to fly in comfort and without trepidation / Cherry Hartman, Julie Sheldon Huffaker.
p.   cm.
Includes index.
ISBN 0-933377-34-7 (lib. bdg). — ISBN 0-933377-33-9 (trade paper)
1. Fear of flying.   I. Huffaker, Julie Sheldon, 1967- .
II. Title.
RC1090.H37   1995
613.6'8—dc20   95–10096

THE EIGHTH MOUNTAIN PRESS
624 Southeast Twenty-ninth Avenue
Portland, Oregon 97214
(503) 233-3936

To Helen, whose love and support make everything possible. —C.H.

To Ruth Huffaker, whose honesty and pluck lend me courage as I spread my own wings. — J.S.H.

TABLE OF CONTENTS

How to Use this Book   13

I. CALMING YOUR FEAR OF FLYING

1. Fear and Control: Letting Go   17

2. Fear of Flying   19

3. How to Focus Your Mind's Eye to Reduce Anxiety   21
Guided Imagery   21
Learning the Technique   22
Active and Passive Relaxation   30
Finding the Right Fantasy   32
Rehearsing a Relaxed Flight   38
The Day of Your Flight   46

4. Knowledge Is Power   47
How the Plane Stays in the Air   47
Weather and Turbulence   51
How U.S. Planes Are Regulated for Safety   53
Inflight Sights, Sounds, and Vibrations   58

5. If You're Still Having a Hard Time   62
Desensitization   62
Therapy   63
Fearful Flyer Programs   63

II. TAKING CHARGE OF YOUR OWN COMFORT

6. Schedule to Avoid Delays   *67*
Air Traffic Patterns   *67*
Crossing Time Zones   *68*
Flight Classification: Connecting, Nonstop, Direct   *69*

7. The ABCs of Seat Selection and Boarding Passes   *71*
Which Seat Is Best?   *71*
Boarding Passes   *79*

8. Strategies for Eating Well   *81*
Ordering Special Meals   *82*
Brown Bagging   *83*

9. Manage Luggage Like an Expert   *87*
Checking Your Luggage   *87*
Traveling with Carry-ons   *90*
Choosing Luggage for Comfort   *92*
Dealing with Damaged, Late, or Lost Luggage   *94*

10. The Advantages of Arriving Early   *98*

11. Navigate Security Checkpoints with Ease   *100*
Film   *102*
Computer Equipment   *102*

12. How to Cope with Changes in Air Pressure   *103*
Ear Pain and Popping   *103*
Swollen Feet   *106*
Sluggish Digestion   *106*
Scheduling Dental Work   *107*
Attention, Divers!   *107*

13. The Truth about the Air up There   *108*
Breathing in a Crowded Space   *108*

Breathing Desert Air   *110*

Coping with Smoking   *113*

Managing Volatile Temperatures   *114*

14. Avoid Backaches   *116*

Posture   *116*

Stretching and Circulation   *120*

15. Escape Noise   *122*

Earplugs   *122*

Headphones   *123*

16. Sleep Soundly   *124*

Getting Comfortable   *124*

Blocking Light and Sound   *126*

Safeguarding Your Sanctity   *127*

17. Prevent Motion Sickness   *128*

A Clash of the Senses   *128*

Staying Comfortable   *129*

Medication Options   *131*

Airbag Etiquette   *133*

18. How to Deal with Difficult Passengers   *134*

Employing Social Cues   *134*

Speaking Your Mind   *136*

If You're Sitting Near Children   *136*

19. Fly Defensively   *138*

20. Know Your Rights   *141*

Delays   *142*

Cancellations   *143*

Overbooking   *144*

21. Make the Most of Your Layovers   *147*

Stashing the Heavies   *147*

Sleuthing Airport Conveniences   *148*
Conducting Business   *152*

22. Avoid Jet Lag   *154*
Your Body's Internal Clock   *154*
Tips for Easier Adjustment   *155*
Method I: Signaling with Melatonin   *156*
Method II: The Anti–Jet Lag Diet   *157*
Anxiety and Attitude   *159*

A Departing Note   *161*

Appendix A: Additional Information for Flyers   *163*
Flying with Children   *163*
Children Flying Solo   *169*
Pregnant Passengers   *170*
Air Travelers with Disabilities   *171*
Traveling with Animals   *175*

Appendix B: Sources for Flight Books and Accessories   *179*

Appendix C: Consumer Flying Publications   *183*

Index   *185*

ACKNOWLEDGMENTS

Generous support and expert participation from a variety of sources helped lift *The Fearless Flyer* off the ground. We would like to thank Amy Schuster, whose idea originally gave birth to this book. We appreciate the women of Ridings Travel Agency for their enthusiasm and for sharing a rich array of travel resources. For his clear and patient explanation of body mechanics, we are grateful to David Deppeler of the Texas Back Institute. And we extend monumental thanks to the pilots and personnel of many airlines for providing detailed answers to our inexhaustible questions.

For their invaluable red ink, we are indebted to our readers: Nichola Zaklan, Kathleen Herron, Ila Suzanne, Anndee Hochman, Janet Howey, and John Rehm. Their feedback was a crucial element in *The Fearless Flyer's* evolution.

Finally, we profess new understanding for the tribute authors often pay their editors. For her tireless editing, her tenacious attention to detail, and the overriding enthusiasm that carried this project to print, we thank ours.

Thank you, Ruth Gundle.

While flying may be the most convenient way to get from here to there, 44 percent of the American public feels apprehensive about stepping aboard a plane. The rest dread the toll that air travel takes on body and temperament. You've picked up *The Fearless Flyer* because you fit into one or both categories, and you want to do something about it. You won't be disappointed. If you follow any part of our advice, your flight experience will be dramatically improved.

Flying is the safest mode of vehicular transportation. No, it's not perfect. But nothing in this world is perfectly safe. While we're all for consumer activism addressing flight safety and comfort, this book is not about that. This book is about what you can do to get the most out of your flight experience right now. Starting today, *you can calm your fear of flying*, and *you can take charge of your own comfort*.

Similarly, take charge of the way you read this book. Don't let us lead you by the nose from beginning to end. Turn first to those sections that are most important to you.

If you're a fearful flyer, start at the beginning. Read and practice the exercises. (Even if you're not a fearful flyer, take a look at Chapter Four, "Knowledge Is Power.")

If you're a discontented flyer, go directly to Part Two. Skip the sections that don't interest you, with one exception: *Everyone* needs to read about dehydration in Chapter Thirteen, "Breathing Desert Air."

Among these pages are tips for savvy travel and information about specific products and resources we recommend. At the end you'll find a list of additional publications that highlight air travel issues, as well as mail-order sources for flight-specific products. Toll-free numbers are for U.S. dialing unless otherwise noted; prices are given in U.S. dollars.

Take *The Fearless Flyer* with you when you go; tuck it in your carry-on for easy reference. Tab the exercises and information you'll want to find quickly. Mark it up, make notes for yourself, and be sure to let us know if you come across new ideas or suggestions for the next edition. We'll be pleased to send you a complimentary copy if we use them.

I

CALMING YOUR
FEAR *of* FLYING

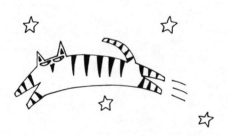

·1·

Fear and Control: Letting Go

Recently a client of Cherry's described his flight from San Francisco to Houston. "As we were approaching the airport, I looked out the window and saw that we were flying above giant towers of storm clouds, with just extraordinary colors and patterns. It was a magnificent sight, and I felt exhilarated until I realized we had to land down there. In fact, we didn't land. We circled for an hour and a half trying to wait out the storm. Finally, the pilot announced we were going on to New Orleans. I calculated that New Orleans was about five hundred miles away and I just knew that after all that time we'd spent circling, we wouldn't have enough fuel to make it. I was terrified. I spent the whole rest of the flight praying and saying good-bye in my head to my family. Other passengers seemed distressed, too. One man threatened to punch out a flight attendant who wouldn't let him go to the bathroom because the Fasten Seatbelt sign was on.

"When we were finally safely on the ground and I was waiting to collect my bags, I started talking to a young woman who had been on the same flight. To my astonishment, she had actually gotten a lot of extra work done on the extended flight, so she viewed it as a bonus. 'Weren't you afraid?' I asked her. 'No,' she said. 'I'm good at what I do. I figure the people flying the plane know what they're doing, so I'm willing to let them be in charge.'"

Many of us have a hard time letting someone else fly the plane. Not that we really want to go through the training and get our own pilot's license. It's just that letting someone else be in control is difficult. For many who lacked competent parenting as children—and had to figure things out for themselves—the world feels scary and unpredictable. We try to make our world "safer" by taking charge and leaving very little to chance. We don't trust that other people will look out for our best interests. Even those who received adequate parenting can regress to earlier developmental stages when under stress and react inappropriately to those in charge.

Fight or flight is our instinctual response to fear, but by the time we're adults, we've been socialized to not run away or hit. So when we are fearful we often become controlling, thinking consciously or unconsciously: *The more I can take charge here, the less scary the situation.*

A person who uses control to manage fear will have a very difficult time in situations where he has very little opportunity to exercise control. Air travel presents one of those situations. A passenger has no responsibility for flying the plane and, unless he requests a tour of the cockpit, will not even come close to the controls. He may have been able to select the seat of his choice but won't have any say over who sits near him. He may have ordered a vegetarian meal but can't know if that will be a baked potato stuffed with cheese and broccoli or a plate of canned peas and a raw carrot.

If you're someone who needs to feel in charge as a way of dealing with fear, learning to be self-aware can make a big difference. For some people, this is a complex process that can be accomplished only with the help of a therapist. Many, however, respond readily to the simple suggestion to pay attention to their inner process and redirect it. You can practice saying to yourself things like: *Oh, now I'm pushing to the front of the line to board the plane because I'm feeling anxious. Stop. Take a deep breath. I don't need to be in control here.*

You can remind yourself that while it may actually have been a survival-oriented response not to trust the adults around you as a child, what was true then is not necessarily true now. Or you can remember that anxiety pushes you back to earlier ways of coping. You may find that simply understanding why you have a hard time being a passive plane passenger is useful.

·2·

Fear of Flying

Thirty million Americans describe themselves as "anxious flyers." For an additional thirty million travelers, the prospect of flying is absolutely terrifying. Statistically, the reality of air travel is reassuring. Flying is nineteen times safer than driving your car through the neighborhood, an act most of us do without thinking. There are more annual fatalities associated with lawnmowers and bathtubs than there are with planes. In terms of *probability*, M.I.T.'s Sloan School of Management has come up with this statistic: You'd have to take a commercial flight every day for the next twenty-nine thousand years before you'd be involved in an airline crash. Nevertheless, a full 44 percent of the American public feels apprehensive about flying.

There's a name for the fear: aerophobia. While phobias have existed as long as people have resided on earth, fear of flying is a twentieth-century affliction. Experts estimate that more people suffer from aerophobia than from any other phobia except fear of public speaking. A wide and colorful range of individuals shares the fear of traveling aloft; Cher, Princess Di, Aretha Franklin, and Muhammed Ali are all rumored to be among those who suffer.

Aerophobia is unique because it combines several fears. Most people who are afraid to fly also fear heights, are claustrophobic, or both. Additionally, some people have an extreme fear of dying, which comes into sharp focus at the thought of flying. (It's normal to be afraid of dying. Almost everyone is to some degree. It is not rational, however, to be more concerned about dying in a plane than in a car when car travel is a much more dangerous activity.)

Fear of flying can also be the result of dwelling on negative feelings while in the plane. Few of us have much free time to just sit and do nothing. If we use the time on the plane to worry about things, we may associate that worry with flying.

Since we weren't born with wings and the air isn't our natural home, humans have a protective mechanism, known as the Moro reflex, designed to prevent us from falling. It is a grasping response to any stimulus that suggests falling. You've probably experienced this clenching feeling when you're falling asleep or looking down from some height. It's natural to have some anxiety about being up in the air. This mild anxiety can build over time and become a phobia. The same is true for mild anxiety about confinement in close spaces. In fact, all phobias become worse as one ages unless they are consciously addressed.

People deal with their aerophobia in all kinds of ways. One man refuses to board a plane without his Hank Aaron baseball card in his wallet. Another picks his flight numbers from numerology charts. One woman expends an extraordinary amount of energy looking out the window during flights, concentrating on keeping her plane in the air. There are tales of passengers who sublimate their fears by having sex on the plane, earning membership in the legendary "Mile-High Club." (We don't recommend it.)

Many people use alcohol or tranquilizers to keep their anxiety in check. While these may seem to help in the short run, they create more problems than they solve. For many people, alcohol increases rather than decreases anxiety; the popular sedatives Xanax and Valium are addictive. Both alcohol and antidepressants hinder the body's adjustment to flight.

Rather than mask your fear, you can quite simply reduce it. The solution is not to make the airplane larger, to fly closer to the ground, to give each passenger more responsibility for the flight, or even to improve the already safe environment of the aircraft. Remember: Fear of flying is irrational. Air travel is the safest form of motorized vehicular transportation. To feel more comfortable as passengers aboard an airplane, we have to transform the fear, not change the reality of the situation.

·3·

How to Focus Your Mind's Eye to Reduce Anxiety

Your body doesn't know the difference between a mental image you create and something you perceive that's "really" happening. So if you conjure up a scene of your plane falling out of the sky your body will activate its emergency fight-or-flight response and pump adrenaline into your muscles to prepare for action. Since the emergency isn't really happening, however, there's nothing to do with all that adrenaline, and you're left feeling jittery. In exactly the same way as you involuntarily conjure up frightening thoughts, you can create positive images. You may have to keep your body strapped into the seat, but your mind can take you to a hammock swinging in a balmy ocean breeze or a leather sofa in front of a blazing fire in a cozy mountain cabin. Or, if you prefer, you can play eighteen holes of perfect golf or hike a woodsy trail or scuba dive off a coral reef.

Guided Imagery

If being on a plane is uncomfortable, *get off*. Not in reality. You've got that important meeting in Cleveland or a rendezvous with an old friend in Paris or the kids are crazy to see Disneyland. You have a good reason to fly. But you don't have to stay on the plane in your mind for the whole trip. Use guided imagery (sometimes called self-hypnosis) to "leave."

The word *hypnosis* can conjure up some scary images of mind control, brain washing, or being on a stage clucking like a chicken. Rest assured—that's not what this is about. While you may never have been formally hypnotized by a hypnotherapist, you've probably had the experience of being under hypnosis thousands of times. Have you ever been reading a book and noticed that you've turned several pages and haven't actually read a word? Or been driving your car and all of a sudden thought, "How'd I get here? I don't remember crossing the bridge." You've been in a trance state. Your teacher probably called it daydreaming when she caught you looking out the window, not paying attention to long division. Hypnosis, trance, daydreaming—it's all the same thing. It's the experience you have right before you fall asleep at night, when you're drifting and thoughts are passing by.

There are three levels of trance: light, medium, and deep. Deep trance is what is always shown in the movies when the person seems almost comatose. Only about one person in ten is capable of deep trance, and that's with a lot of practice. The rest of us will experience a light or medium trance in which we'll still be aware of noises around us. They just won't bother us.

Research has shown that a light trance is just as effective as a deep one for relaxing, learning new skills, and giving ourselves positive messages. Most people experience different levels throughout a short hypnotic experience. They will go from feeling deep into the trance to floating close to the surface of awareness.

There are a lot of myths about hypnosis. One of them is that dumb people are easier to hypnotize. Actually, the opposite is true. Anyone who is able to concentrate is able to hypnotize herself. The greater your ability to concentrate the easier it is. You can improve your ability to concentrate with practice.

Learning the Technique

Read through this section as many times as you need to get the idea and then practice the exercises. Suspend your critical faculties and imagine a melodious, deep voice reading to you. These exercises will work better with your eyes closed.

Some people find it easier to learn the guided imagery

technique or to practice it if they hear, rather than read the instructions. You can read the text into a tape recorder and then play the tape when you want to do the exercises. If you get hung up on the sound of your own voice—and a lot of people do—ask someone else to read the instructions into a tape recorder for you. Once you are familiar with the routine you will probably find that you can do them without the need of a recording.

There is no danger in self-hypnosis. If at any time you become uncomfortable or need to attend to something, simply stop.

▪ **Make certain your arms and legs aren't crossed.** If they are, they may fall asleep, as you won't be moving them for a few minutes.

▪ **Take a couple of deep breaths.** Draw the air deep into your body so that your belly rises as you inhale and deflates as you let the air go. Exhale slowly and completely. (Focus on the exhale and the inhale will follow automatically.) Breathing this way slows your heartbeat, lowers your blood pressure and relaxes your body.

▪ **You may hear sounds or noises during this time.** They are not important and you do not need to attend to them. If something important happens you'll know it.

▪ **Count slowly backwards from five to one.** As you count, see yourself moving down in some safe, comfortable way. Walk down a staircase or a path to the beach or take an escalator down. Use an image that's particularly soothing to you. It can be along a river, in a field, amid Roman ruins. Play around until you find the right one for you.

▪ **When you reach one, set your internal alarm clock** for however long you want to stay in this relaxed place: three minutes, thirty minutes, two hours, however long you want. (Have you ever had the experience of not setting an alarm clock but instead telling yourself you want to wake up at seven o'clock and you do? That's your internal alarm clock.) If you've never done it before, don't worry. It's easy and it's something you get better at with practice. If you've closed your eyes, just tell yourself to open them in twenty minutes.

Once you've set the time, you can stop worrying about it. When the time is up you'll open your eyes and feel refreshed and relaxed, as though you've had a short nap.

While you're in this relaxed state you can do whatever you want to do. You can take yourself in fantasy any place you want to be. You can do in fantasy anything you want to do. Or you can simply clear your mind of all thoughts and enjoy the refreshing blankness of not thinking. Or you can give yourself messages that would be good for you to hear like, "It's okay, you're doing fine, relax."

Practice Using Your Imagination

To take yourself places in fantasy, you need to be able to see pictures, hear sounds, smell scents, and feel sensations. Try this out: Look at the list of objects named below and let yourself see them in your mind. If you don't see them, or you see something else, don't worry about it, just go on. Allow a few minutes to practice these.

Cat

Tree

House

Duck

Pond

Apple

Yellow apple

Green apple

Red apple

Now try some sounds. Let yourself hear them:

Whistle of a wind

Roar of the ocean

Footsteps

Whinny of a horse

Crackle of a campfire

Now try some smells:

Smoke from a campfire

A rose

An orange

Vinegar

Hot apple pie fresh from the oven

Now try feeling some sensations:

Wind ruffling your hair

Sun on your face

Running your hand across moss

A splash of cold water

Someone's hand in yours

You probably noticed that you could more easily access one sense than another. By going through all of them, the ones you're good at will help you to develop the ones that are more difficult. For example, if you have trouble smelling the smoke from a campfire, try seeing the flames or hearing the crackle. You will find that it will eventually lead you to the smell. Once you get the hang of it, try going someplace in fantasy.

Imagine you're on an ocean beach. Look around you and notice all the colors you see, the tans and grays and whites of the sand; the blues and greens and whites of the ocean and the blues and whites and silvers of the sky.

Hear the waves lapping against the sand and the cry of sea gulls.

Smell the scent of salt and seaweed.

Feel the ocean breeze moving across your face and through your hair.

Feel the penetrating warmth of the sun on your head and face and shoulders.

Now take yourself someplace that's part of your own imaginary landscape, whether it's a place you've been and loved or a place you've wholly imagined.

Notice what you see, what you hear, what you smell, and what you feel.

When you're ready, come back.

Now try *doing* something in fantasy. Go back to the ocean.

Imagine yourself running along the beach.

Feel the sand give way beneath your feet.

Feel the muscles of your legs working.

Feel your arms swinging.

Feel your heart pumping.

Feel the sun on your skin.

Feel the wind blowing on your face.

Feel your lungs taking in huge gulps of air.

When you've had enough, stop.

Now do something in your own imaginary landscape and really feel your body doing it.

It can be as simple as a leisurely walk along a path in the woods or as active as swimming on a quiet lake.

Feel the sensations on the surface of your body, the smells, the air, the temperature, etc.

And feel what's going on inside: your heartbeat, your muscles, your breathing.

Practice Emptying Your Mind

Now clear your mind of all thoughts and enjoy the refreshing stillness of not thinking. Focus on your breathing. Don't try to change it. Just notice your breath going in and out. You may find that thoughts tend to come in. If they do, gently return your awareness to your breathing. Some people find it helpful to focus on a single word or sound. You could use the word *peace* if you want. Just repeat the word or sound over and over again. If other thoughts stray in just whisk them away as though you were using a broom or a scarf and go back to the word or sound that you've chosen.

Practice Giving Yourself Positive Messages

Finally, practice giving yourself messages that would be good for you to hear. These are sometimes called affirmations. For example: "Relax. You're doing a very good job. You don't have to work so hard. It's okay." Or, "I am feeling relaxed and easy. I'm confident I can do whatever I need to. I can afford to let down and be easy." Either the "you" or the "I" voice is okay to use, whichever feels more natural to you.

If a negative image slips through, "correct" it by crossing it out, literally draw a line or an X through the image and then replace it with a positive one, such as your plane gliding to a smooth landing at your destination.

Active and Passive Relaxation

If you're having trouble relaxing in preparation for doing the guided imagery it may be because you need an active route to relaxation rather than a passive one. Some people relax best by just letting themselves go limp and enjoy napping or reading quietly. Others find that kind of stillness very hard to achieve and prefer to relax by doing something active: running, playing tennis, gardening, etc. If you're more suited to active rather than passive relaxation, try progressive body relaxation or deep breathing.

Progressive Body Relaxation

Follow these suggestions with your eyes open. Once you become practiced at it, you can do it with your eyes closed.

Take a couple of **deep breaths.**

Start with your **toes** and clench the muscles tight. Hold them for just a moment and then let them go, relax them.

Now, do the same thing with the rest of your **foot,** the ball and the arch and the heel. Tighten them. Then, let them go.

Do the same with your **calf** muscles, pull them tight. Hold them. Let them go.

Now, the muscles of your **thighs**. Tighten them. And relax them. Let them go.

Do the same with the muscles of your **hips**. Pull them tight. And relax them. Let them go.

Now, do the same thing with the muscles of your **stomach** and **abdomen**. Tighten them. Relax them.

Do the same with the **small of your back**. Tighten the muscles. Let them go.

Now, your **upper back**, tighten the muscles. Relax them.

Do the same thing with the muscles of your **chest.** Tighten them. And relax them.

Do the same with your **hands** and **arms**. Tighten your hands into fists. Relax them.

Now, your **shoulders.** Pull them up so they're touching your earlobes. Relax them, let them fall back down.

Tighten the muscles of your **scalp** and **forehead.** Relax them.

Do the same with the muscles around your **eyes,** squeeze them tight. And let them go.

And finally, tighten the muscles of your **jaw** and **mouth.** Make a scary face. And let it go.

Take a moment to see if you're still holding any muscles tight. If so, and you want to relax them, picture them in your mind's eye as relaxing, becoming loose and limp. And then *feel* them relaxing, becoming loose and limp.

Now begin counting backwards from five to one.

Deep Breathing

Take a **deep breath** all the way into your stomach, allowing it to fill like a balloon.

Hold the breath for a count of three and then blow it out, blowing out tension with the breath.

Pause a moment and take another deep breath.

Do this five to ten times until you are feeling very relaxed.

Finding the Right Fantasy

It's important to find a fantasy that you can really imagine yourself in. Read over the following scenarios to see if one calls to you. If not, experiment until you develop one that works for you. You may want to use different fantasies at different times or continually tinker with the ones you use.

Country Meadow

Imagine you're in a country meadow on an early summer day. Look around you and notice all the colors you see. The greens of the grasses, the blues, yellows, pinks and reds of the wildflowers, the blues and whites of the sky. It's a beautiful day; there's nothing you have to do and nothing you have to think about. There's a woods on the other side of the meadow. You might enjoy walking through the meadow to stroll among the trees. If you do, you'll feel the swish of grasses against your legs as you walk. Hear the calls of birds and the hum and whir of insects. Feel the warmth of the sun on your face and head and shoulders. A slight breeze brushes your face and ruffles your hair. Smell the scent of grasses and wildflowers. Your body feels loose and comfortable as you walk. *There's nothing you have to do and nothing you have to think about.*

As you get closer to the woods you begin to smell pine and cedar. Soon, you enter the forest. It's a little cooler here, but the sun still filters through the trees and you can still feel its warmth on your face, the top of your head, and shoulders. Hear the crunch of pine needles beneath your feet as you walk and the calls of birds. You can also hear the sound of rushing water—there's a creek nearby and you're walking toward it. The sound grows louder and soon you can see the clear water tumbling over rocks and pebbles. There are some boulders near the edge of the creek. You can sit on one if you'd like. It's warm enough, and if you want to you can take off your shoes and socks and dangle your feet in the water. Feel the coolness of the water on your feet, contrasting with the warmth of the sun on your head, face and shoulders. It's a very pleasant place to be. *There's nothing you have to do or think about.* You can stay as long as you like and explore as much of this landscape as you want.

Nurturing Person

Imagine you're in the woods following a path. Smell the scent of pine. Hear the calls of birds. Your body feels loose and comfortable as you walk. Your arms swing rhythmically. The path begins to seem familiar. You realize that it leads to a house in the woods where a very nurturing person lives who will be very glad to see you. Soon you can see the house. It's a clapboard structure. Climb the steps to the porch and knock on the door. The nurturing person answers. *You take the fantasy from here. If you draw a blank here's one way it might go:*

The nurturing person greets you with a warm smile and a hug. She invites you in, and you choose a comfortable overstuffed chair. She's just put the kettle on for tea and you hear it whistling in the kitchen. She returns in a few minutes with a tray that holds a flowered teapot and two cups. As the tea steeps, she asks you about what's been happening in your life. You tell her. She listens very attentively and offers supportive responses. When you finish she takes your hand and looks into your eyes and tells you how very well you are handling the challenges life is offering you. She gives you a cup of tea; you drink the most delicious beverage you've ever tasted. Your tongue explores a lingering hint of cinnamon and cloves. You're feeling very calm and relaxed and very comforted. After a while she suggests a walk in her garden. She leads you out the back door into a world of flowers and plum and pear trees. A path winds, creating garden "rooms." The final one has bushes covered with delicately scented, white blossoms surrounding a small pool. She tells you it is a healing mineral pool and invites you to bathe. She lifts the lid of a small bench and pulls out a thick, white towel that smells of cedar. She leaves. You undress, slip into the warm water, and soak away all your cares, aches and pains.

A Safe Place

Imagine creating a room that will be totally safe and comfortable for you. It might be in your home or it could be someplace else, but it will be only for you and just as you would like it. You don't have to consider anyone else's needs. Think about the dimensions of the room. Is it square, oblong, round, oval, or some combination of these? Is the ceiling high or low? Are there windows? What do you see when you look out the windows? Are the walls plastered, wood paneled, logs, stucco? What color are the walls? What about the floor? Is it hardwood, carpeted? Are there area rugs? Put some furniture in the room. Sofa? Chairs? Bed? Chaise? Does the room have a fireplace or wood stove? Are there paintings? Pottery? Books? Plants? Fill it with everything you need for your comfort or aesthetic pleasure. Now put yourself in your room. What are you wearing? *Notice what you see, what you hear, what you smell and what you feel.* Allow yourself to change anything at anytime—it is your room. Come here whenever you feel worried, anxious or are in need of comforting.

Body Massage

Imagine lying on your stomach on a massage table. There is an opening in the table through which your face fits that allows you to lie in perfect alignment. Melodic music plays. You take a couple of deep breaths as a masseuse begins to apply warm, fragrant oil to your back. He smooths the oil all across the length and breadth of your back with firm, easing strokes. You feel very relaxed. Next, he stands in front of your head and massages your shoulders. He gently pulls your right arm up, massages it and replaces it next to your body. He does the same with your left arm. Now he stands at your feet and massages your legs, beginning with the thighs and working down to your ankles. Then he begins to work on your feet. Massaging each toe, then the ball, instep, and heel. Your feet feel wonderfully alive and tingly with pleasant energy. Now it's time for you to roll over. The masseuse works on your neck, soothing away any tightness. He massages your scalp and gently strokes your face. He leaves the room and you lie there feeling content and peaceful.

White Light

Some people use a white light to create a sense of safety. (Feel free to choose any color: golden, rosy, etc.) You can put this light around yourself anytime you choose. You can also send it to someone else, someone you want to protect or someone who isn't feeling well and needs some extra healing energy. When you're traveling you can put a white or colored light around your car, train, or plane.

Here's how: Imagine a bright light coming from—*fill in the blank:* The Goddess, God, the sky, the universal source of all power, the source of all creation, or whatever image fits with your spirituality. The light comes directly through the top of your head and slowly descends, filling your entire head, brain, eyes, nose, ears, mouth and throat with healing energy. It continues flowing down your body, down your neck into your shoulders, arms, hands, relaxing and healing as it flows. All the way down your spine, down through your chest, flowing through the valves and passages of your heart, into your lungs, filling them with a powerful healing energy. Feel it go down into your abdomen, through each of your organs, your stomach, liver, kidneys, etc. The light continues into your legs, feet, toes. Then the light comes back to your heart, exits your body and completely surrounds the surface of your body. Now project the light to surround the entire surface of the plane with the bright, protective light. Within the light, no harm can come.

Rehearsing a Relaxed Flight

Have you ever had the experience of walking into a room and being engulfed by feelings that seem to come right out of the smell of the furniture polish, the old davenport, or lentil soup simmering on the stove? Or while walking down a path in autumn, suddenly remembering vividly one day twenty-five years earlier when you leaped into a pile of leaves with your best friend? The light, the colors, the feel of the air— bring forth not just the memory, but the feelings you felt at the time.

It's also possible to *consciously* attach positive feeling to specific "triggers." That's what you will be doing when you rehearse a relaxed flight. You will be establishing a connection between feeling relaxed and going through the motions of arriving at the airport and getting on the plane. You will find that, with practice, your former feelings of anxiety will be replaced with feeling calm.

We'll use two "anchor points" to remind you that you're feeling calm and relaxed: going through airport and airplane doorways and putting your feet flat on the floor. The latter can be used at any time to reestablish feelings of calm.

As soon as you know you're going to be flying, and you begin to worry about it, start to prepare for a fearless flight. It's helpful to get the itinerary from your travel agent so you'll know all the takeoffs and landings. Rehearsing is as important as packing the right clothes.

- **Choose a quiet space** where you won't be interrupted.

- **Turn the phone off.**

- **Sit in a comfortable chair.** You may lie down if you choose. However, if you tend to fall asleep easily, sitting is better. Make sure neither your arms nor your legs are crossed; they may fall asleep if they are.

- **Read through the instructions** as often as necessary, then close your eyes. If you prefer to hear, rather than read the instructions, you can read them (or have someone else read them) into a tape recorder.

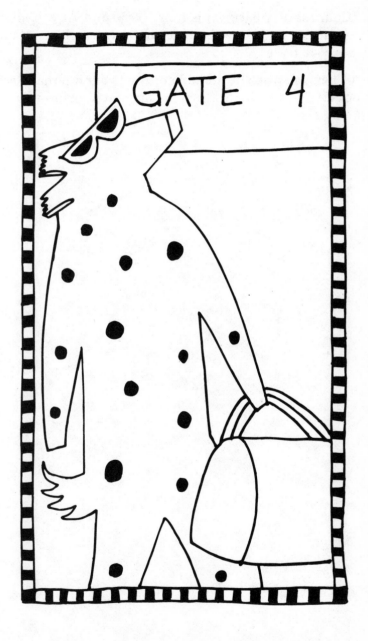

Take a couple of deep breaths. Then exhale fully and completely.

Count slowly backwards from five to one. As you count, see yourself going down in some safe, easy way, like walking down a staircase.

When you reach the number one, set your internal alarm clock for twenty minutes. That's about how long this exercise should take.

Imagine it is the day of your trip.

You awaken from a deep and restful sleep feeling energetic and peaceful and eager to get on with your day.

See yourself going through your morning routine.

Then jump ahead until it's time to go to the airport. See yourself arriving at the airport.

As you go through the door, let it be a reminder that you're feeling calm, comfortable, relaxed.

The doorway is an anchor point. Each time you go through a doorway at the airport, or into the plane itself, it will remind you, you're feeling *calm, comfortable, relaxed, in charge.*

See yourself in line at the check-in counter.

Check your luggage if you wish and proceed to the proper gate.

In the waiting area, choose a seat and let the chair fully support your weight. Take a moment to put your feet flat on the floor, close your eyes, and take a couple of deep breaths.

Notice the contact your feet are making with the floor; let this be a reminder that you're feeling *calm and comfortable.* (Placing your feet flat on the floor is another anchor point; besides, it's good for your body.)

Feel your hands and whatever they're touching. Be aware of their warmth. Feel whatever they're touching, touching you back.

Relax until it's time to board.

See yourself walking down the boarding ramp and going through the portal of the plane.

As you do, remind yourself that you're feeling *calm and confident*.

Find your seat. Stow away your carry-ons and sit down, taking care to place both feet flat on the floor.

Close your eyes and take a couple of deep breaths. Notice the contact your feet are making with the floor. Let this be a reminder that you're feeling *calm and comfortable*.

If at any time you notice yourself becoming anxious, put both feet flat on the floor, close your eyes and take a couple of deep breaths. Remember that you don't have to think about anything, you don't have to do anything. Your job is simply to relax and let the time pass away.

You may want to put a protective light around the plane. Imagine a bright light coming in through the top of your head, completely filling your body with healing energy, and exiting through your heart. Then surround the entire surface of your body with the protective light. Finally, project the light to completely surround the surface of the plane. Within the light, no harm can come.

See yourself sitting comfortably on the plane.

It has been cleared for takeoff and begins moving down the runway, picking up speed and finally lifts into the air.

You're feeling *calm and comfortable.* You're allowing the flight crew to do their job. Your only job is to continue to relax.

You can do whatever you want to. You can read, listen to music, converse with your seat mate, or sleep.

Or you can take yourself in fantasy anywhere you want to be and do in fantasy anything you want to do.

Or you can simply clear your mind of all thoughts or give yourself messages that would be good for you to hear.

See yourself at the end of the flight.

You're sitting comfortably in your seat as the captain announces the descent. You've put away your tray table and returned your seat to its upright position.

Take a moment to put your feet flat on the floor, close your eyes, and take a couple of deep breaths. Congratulate yourself on a job well done.

You've been successful in remaining relaxed and this portion of your trip is nearly completed.

Move ahead to the point where the plane touches down and continues down the runway and finally rolls to a stop.

Stand up, collect your belongings and walk up the aisle and through the portal of the plane. As you do, congratulate yourself again on a job well done.

Continue this rehearsal for the next leg of your journey.

The Day of Your Flight

From the time you wake up in the morning until you arrive at the airport, go through your routine with a deliberate calm, concentrating on moving slowly. Remember the anchors you've established in your rehearsals:

- As you go through the door of the airport, remind yourself that you're feeling **calm.**

- While sitting in the waiting area, place your feet flat on the floor and remind yourself that you're feeling **relaxed.**

You may want to use headphones to listen to the instructions you've prerecorded or enjoy soothing music as you do the exercises.

- When you go through the jetway door, remind yourself that you're feeling **easy.**

- When you go through the door to the plane, remind yourself that you're feeling **confident.**

- When you take your seat, place your feet flat on the floor and remind yourself that you're feeling **in charge.**

Put a light around the plane if you wish.

- During takeoff, close your eyes, put your feet flat on the floor, take a couple of deep breaths, and remind yourself that you're feeling **peaceful.**

During the flight, if at any time you feel anxious, do the relaxation techniques you have learned. Use your favorite fantasy or make up a new one. Eyeshades may be helpful. Not only will they block out light, but they may signal other people to leave you alone.

- As the pilot prepares for landing, again close your eyes, put your feet flat on the floor, take a couple of deep breaths, and remind yourself that you're feeling **comfortable.**

- As you go through the door on your way out of the plane, congratulate yourself on a job well done. You have remained **relaxed** throughout the flight.

·4·

Knowledge Is Power

As humans, we are naturally suspicious of what we don't understand. One way to reduce apprehension about air travel is to know how it works. How do planes stay up in the air? What is turbulence, and when is it dangerous? Once you're buckled in and under way, what's going on? *And what are all those noises?*

How the Plane Stays in the Air

At 10:35 A.M. on a windy December day in 1903, bicycle mechanic Orville Wright became the first human to sustain powered flight. He lay down in the wood and canvas aircraft and rose above a sandy beach along the Outer Banks of North Carolina. Orville stayed aloft for twelve seconds; he traveled 120 feet, less than the length of a modern commercial jet.

"Damned if they ain't flew!" was the comment of one bystander. Many people still have the same mystified reaction. How could a commercial airplane weighing 600,000 pounds, the equivalent of 34.2 fully matured male African elephants or 15,000 well-packed suitcases, stay up in the air?

Principle 1: Lift

The answer is simpler than you might think. Try this: The next time you're in a car (it's best to run this experiment as a passenger), roll your window down and hold your arm out straight. Flatten your palm and fingers so that the palm faces down, parallel to the asphalt. Feel the air hitting the front of your arm? Now try cupping your hand, and tilt your arm gently so that the front side of your hand, where the thumb is, rises slightly. You should feel a substantial lift driving your palm up into the air. Lift is affected by the angle of your hand—or an aircraft's wing—as it meets oncoming air. The faster you're going, the less angle you need to produce the same amount of lift.

How does that plane stay in the air? A higher curve on the top surface of the wing makes air passing over the arched surface travel farther than the air that passes underneath; although the same amount of air passes above and below, the air above is stretched out over a longer space. The high-pressure air below each wing—high pressure generated by the shape of the wing itself—holds the aircraft aloft.

Imagine two boxes, both containing the same amount of air. Stretch the edges of one box. The air inside spreads out to fill the additional area, and the density of the air in that box becomes less. The air *above* the wing, therefore, is *less dense*. Where density is less, air pressure is lower. The air passing *underneath* the wing is *higher* in pressure. That air, therefore, *creates upward force*—and a lot of it. The wing span on a Boeing 767 is wider than a ten-lane highway.

If you find it hard to believe that air moving over the top of an object can cause it to rise, try it for yourself. Hold two corners on the same side of a piece of paper—any old notepad or copier variety—with the thumb and forefinger of each hand. Bring the edge of the paper to your mouth, just beneath your lower lip. The paper will hang limp. Blow. Does the far edge rise? Your exhale is decreasing the pressure of the air above it. The air underneath, now higher in pressure, exerts upward force and lifts the page. This principle of *lift* accounts for one-third of the flying equation.

Principle 2: Thrust

Just as air flow over the wings generates lift, air flow over the vigorously turning blades of a propeller produces forward motion, or thrust. (The change in air pressure below the wing of an airplane creates *upward* force, while the change in air

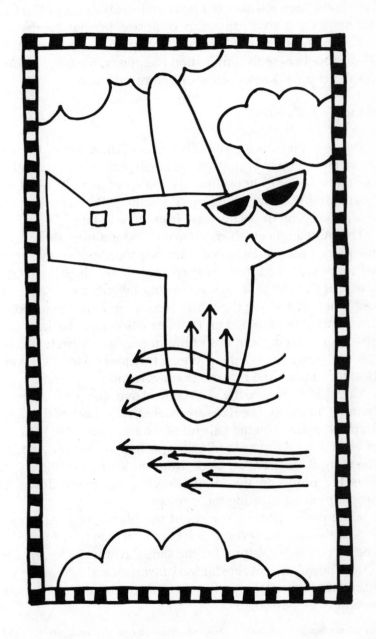

pressure behind the blades of a propeller creates *forward* force.) The effect is the same you experience when blowing up a balloon, then release your hold on its rubber neck. The balloon flies off in a direction opposite to that of the air whooshing out. Today's commercial planes combine modified propellers with combustion engines in the large, drumlike jet engines found below or before each wing.

Principle 3: Control

Control refers to the stabilization and direction of the aircraft. Have you ever noticed the small, flat shelf at the tail of the plane looking almost like an extra set of wings? Called the horizontal stabilizer, this piece balances the action of the wings, keeping the plane level from nose to tail.

The mild angle at which the wings extend from the side of the plane keeps us balanced from side to side. If you've got a window seat, you may be surprised to see the downward curve of the wings straighten during takeoff. In the air, you can look out and see the wings flexing up and down. Don't worry; they're supposed to. That flex works just like the shock absorbers on your car, absorbing impact and vibration. The flex and movement of the wings, sometimes up to fifteen vertical feet, makes the ride easier on you and the aircraft.

Movable flaps give the pilot control over the plane and determine direction. The flaps are located at the back of the horizontal stabilizer, on the tail end of the rudder, and to the rear of each wing. During landing, in particular, you may notice the wing flaps lift at an angle from the surface of the wing. This technique creates drag, slowing the plane down in preparation for meeting the runway.

Some passengers worry about the plane "tipping over." Would the aircraft become unbalanced if everyone formed a line on one side, waiting for the same lavatory? The answer is no. The air currents are far too powerful, and a commercial jet too monumental a craft to be affected by the sum of the weight of its passengers.

For greater detail about the nuts and bolts of commercial airplanes, look for Todd Gold and Ed Sternstein's *From Takeoff to Landing: Everything You Wanted to Know About Airplanes but Had No One to Ask* (Pocket Books, 1991, 112 pages, $8).

Weather and Turbulence

Although the mechanics of flight are not so hard to understand, it's difficult to conceptualize the environment in which all this flying takes place. Earth and water are palpable. We recognize their landscapes. We're used to stomping along on solid earth. We know what it is to push the weight of water behind a crawl stroke, or let it lift us as we float. Air, on the other hand, seems to belong in a completely different category. We don't often "touch" air. It's hard to imagine how we might see it. The truth is that air has mass, harbors current and force, and carries temperature. Planes fly the landscape of the air the way fish navigate water.

When your plane seems to leap to the side, or "fall," it has simply encountered an air pocket. An air pocket isn't a gap or hole—it's a bubble of air riding along at a higher or lower pressure. Although most passengers find it hard to believe, a plane flying through the worst-feeling turbulence doesn't usually register a change in altitude—most shifts are too slight to show up on the instrument panels. Pilots work hard to avoid thunderstorms and turbulent air; not necessarily because the disruptive air is dangerous, but because it's unpleasant for passengers. There are three main types of turbulence: convective air, "weather," and clear air turbulence.

Convection

Convection is the up and down transfer of atmospheric properties like heat (high pressure) and cold (low pressure). The warm air that is always rising off the earth's surface causes convective air turbulence, which is why takeoffs and landings are often bumpy. Mountains and tall buildings located near airports can also affect wind conditions and create convective air turbulence.

Weather

Weather includes warm fronts, cold fronts, changing air masses, and cloud activity—the stuff of the evening news. It may not be comfortable to fly through, but it's seldom hazardous. Flight planners, air traffic controllers, and pilots all study weather readings to chart the smoothest route for passengers.

Lightning, incidentally, is not dangerous to an airplane or its passengers. Even in the event of a direct hit, the plane will not be disabled. Nor can lightning make its way inside the aircraft, to the engine, or to the fuel tanks; the plane's metal skin is engineered to a thickness that prevents this. Planes, in fact, are often struck by lightning. (On average, each plane is hit once every two years.) The lightning traverses the length of the aircraft—which is a nongrounded metal conductor—and exits via a static wick at the tail, built explicitly for this purpose. The static wick discharges electricity as the surge passes through. A small burn mark at the initial point of contact is the lightning's greatest effect.

Passengers often express another weather-related concern: What does it mean if the ground crew is de-icing your plane the moment before takeoff? In winter weather, this is standard procedure. Ice on the wings or tail during takeoff can disturb air flow. A liquid spray, usually a heated solution of glycol and water, is applied to the plane at the gate or the end of the runway. If your plane rolls back to the gate for additional de-icing, it's probably because it's been stuck in line on the runway and needs a refresher. Once the plane is flying, ice is not a factor. The wings provide their own anti-icing device (electrical heat, or hot air) as needed. At cruising altitude, basic chemistry provides another solution: solids sublimate in the extreme cold, bypassing the liquid stage and changing directly to gas.

Also ranking high among passengers' concerns are "wind shears." The term describes a change in winds, often associated with thunderstorms, which can be problematic during landings. Air currents racing downward move out in opposite directions once they reach the ground. The plane hits the headwinds first and is buoyed up, then abruptly hits tailwinds which reduce loft. The plane must climb quickly to maintain the proper trajectory for landing. A pilot's first and primary method of handling wind shears is to avoid them. Pilots monitor thunderstorm locations through information from route planners, air traffic controllers, and their own onboard weather tracking devices. They receive extensive simulator training for direct contact with wind shears but report encountering them in far fewer than 1 percent of all flights.

Clear Air Turbulence

Clear air turbulence is the turbulence that happens when the sky looks open and blue but rapid pressure, temperature, or wind changes are forecasted. If your seatbelt sign stays lit an abnormally long time, it may be that the flight crew is being cautious and wants to keep passengers seated in case the ride gets bumpy. The crew is on the lookout for turbulence caused by abrupt changes in air pressure not yet visible as "weather."

Planes and control towers use instruments that track weather and "see" through clouds. Aircraft are extraordinarily well equipped to handle the pitch and roll of turbulence. When you do hit agitated air, remember the plane will soon pass beyond it; in most cases, pilots are able to move through rough patches in three to four minutes. What feels dramatic and frightening for passengers is usually the high-altitude equivalent of a short gravel patch under the wheels of a Range Rover.

How U.S. Planes Are Regulated for Safety

The U.S. has one of the most stringent regulatory agencies in the world, overseeing more than twenty-five million flights of paying passengers to domestic destinations every year. For information about the regulatory bodies governing international travel scheduled on non-U.S. airlines, or not originating in the United States, consult your travel agent. But keep in mind that although regulatory effectiveness varies from country to country, there's no country in which driving is statistically safer than flying.

TIP If you are concerned about the safety of flying outside the U.S. on a non-U.S. airline, call the State Department's traveler's advisory center (202/647-5225), or its automated fax service (202/647-3000). If a general country warning is appropriate, you'll find it here.

In the United States, air travel is regulated by the Federal Aviation Administration (FAA), whose primary goal is the safety of passengers. The FAA is responsible for airport management, air traffic control, and all air safety and technical matters. They supervise the activities of passengers, pilots, technicians, and on down the line.

The three people in the cockpit at the front of your plane are all pilots, though each takes a different "position"—captain, first officer, or second officer—on any given flight. Pilots must have at least two thousand hours of experience in the air, and pass a battery of tests, before they are considered for hire as commercial pilots. Once hired by a commercial airline, a pilot will go through rigorous training, written and oral exams, simulator and airplane check rides, and at least twenty-five hours of FAA-supervised flying time on the style of aircraft they'll be flying. A pilot must go through this training and testing regimen to fly each type of airplane.

Flight attendants are not just glorified waiters but have undergone between six and twelve weeks of full-time study and are required to spend a certain number of hours in ongoing training each year. The earliest "hostesses" of post–World War I airlines, in fact, were all registered nurses. And strong ones—they loaded passenger luggage, fueled the plane, mended aircraft punctures, and even helped push the craft out of its hangar.

Today, flight attendants are well schooled in emergency procedures and take their responsibilities seriously. By enforcing safety precautions, they play a critical role in ensuring passenger safety. Does that soft-sided duffel bag have to fit *all the way* under the seat? Yes, so no one stumbles on the way out of a row, particularly in the event of an emergency. Do the seatbacks have to come up? Yes, also for ease of passage. Seatbelts? Crucial for protecting jostled passengers from serious injury. The FAA makes sure that there is at least one flight attendant for every fifty seats, empty or full. Most crews fly with more.

Preflight Planning

About two hours before scheduled takeoff, the FAA-licensed dispatchers who work for each airline are busy planning your flight. Their overall criteria are safety, passenger comfort, and economy—*in that order*. Dispatchers evaluate all the possible variables, including weather conditions, route, optimal cruising altitude and speed, and necessary fuel load.

The route is determined by examining the forecasts of an in-house meteorological department as well as that of the U.S. National Weather Service, and taking radar scans, aircraft reports, and satellite photos into account. Cruising altitude (the altitude at which the plane will spend most of its travel time) is selected based on weather, wind, and type of plane. Most commercial planes cruise at around thirty-five thousand feet, just above the earth's lower troposphere layer. The troposphere is where most clouds form and weather happens. Above this layer, the temperature is usually constant so there's no real wind or weather.

Cruising speed, the rate the plane will travel once it has reached cruising altitude, is figured by balancing the fastest possible flying time with the most economical amount of fuel to carry. Commercial jets average five hundred miles per hour for most of their route.

For many passengers, flight anxiety manifests itself as worry over fuel load. Rest assured. There's more than enough onboard. Every plane leaves the airport with "trip fuel" to see it safely to its scheduled destination, enough extra to accommodate anticipated delays or rerouting, one or two hours' worth of "hold fuel" for unexpected holdups, and an FAA-required minimum of forty-five minutes' reserve. Total fuel level is monitored constantly from the cockpit.

After your plane's route, altitude, speed, fuel load, and alternate paths have been determined, a dispatcher will coordinate this overall flight plan with air traffic control. When the FAA's central computer in Washington, D.C., approves it, the flight plan is filed electronically so the instant the pilot logs on radar, that plan is accessible to all the air traffic control towers who watch over the flight.

Mechanical Checks

You're at the gate, relaxed and sitting with both feet on the floor. You've got one arm draped over a pile of carry-ons, and you're waiting to hear the airline agent's call for boarding.

"Did you hear?" says the guy in the gray business suit and wildly colored tie. "Mechanical delay." He pops a handful of corn nuts in his mouth and rolls his eyes. "As long as they don't send us off without an engine!"

What this fellow doesn't know is that the FAA has a rigorous and efficient inspection system. An in-service mechanic meets every flight. Most of the time, repair needs are anticipated through a careful monitoring of the plane's mechanical log book. The FAA requires, in fact, that airplanes and their engines undergo strictly scheduled maintenance overhauls—far more frequently than the average automobile—even if the aircraft has an absolutely spotless bill of health.

When a crew member notices a mechanical problem of any kind, a report is radioed in before the plane touches down. If this problem affects the safety of the flight in any way, the mechanic meeting the flight will bring parts for replacement. If the part can't be replaced in a timely manner, another aircraft will be substituted.

Most often, the mechanic meeting the flight has no adjustments to make. She proceeds straight to the walk-around, making the first of two preflight inspections that will take place before the plane heads back out to the runway. She checks the exterior of the plane, and then comes into the cockpit for a look at the instruments and internal fluid levels. When the mechanic is satisfied that the plane is completely air worthy, she signs the log book and gives the okay for passengers to board.

As soon as the mechanic has finished her inspection, the pilot or copilot checks more than a hundred items on the exterior and in the cockpit of the plane. Fuel line, landing gear, brakes, gauges—there's a lot of ground to cover. The Boeing 767, at 180 feet, is almost the length of a football field, and the highest point on the aircraft is about five stories tall. While the pilot makes his rounds, there is a flurry of activity around the aircraft. Your suitcase moves up a conveyor belt loading baggage and cargo. The fuel and catering trucks pull close. A third truck refills drinking water while another siphons off lavatory waste. It all happens at once, in the thirty minutes before your plane is scheduled to lift off. When your plane passes inspection and all preparations for the journey are complete, a gate agent will welcome you for boarding.

Air Traffic Control

At one time, the laws of the sky were vague. There was no such thing as air traffic control. Pilots embraced the "see and avoid" theory of air traffic management. (We have tremendous visibility, they reasoned, we'll just see the other planes and avoid them.) They believed in the "big sky concept." (It's a big sky; what are the odds?) The chances of sharing airspace with another plane were fairly remote. Today, however, the scenario is radically different. Hundreds of thousands of planes pass through airports each day—more than 2,200 through Chicago O'Hare International Airport alone.

The orderly, carpeted air traffic control tower is walled in glass and equipped with the latest weather monitors, radar screens, and maplike digital displays. There is a cup of coffee here, a glass of water there, but no real distractions. Although they have chairs, controllers usually remain standing on the job. To balance the intensity, air traffic controllers get frequent half-hour breaks—three or four per eight-hour shift.

Air traffic controllers know their airport, moment-by-moment air conditions, and the specific takeoff and landing requirements of each plane type. They identify each plane by its electronic "tag," following it across a variety of digital maps and screens. Through headsets, controllers maintain direct verbal contact with the pilots and each other. Their average exchange is three to four seconds, the language of communication precise and well practiced.

There is at least one air traffic controller assigned to each tier of the airspace for which the tower is responsible. Controllers even monitor the landing conditions at your plane's destination airport, and, if there are complications on the receiving end, may keep you from departing (far less expensive—and nerve-wracking—than circling over a fogged-in landing strip).

About fifteen minutes before your plane is ready to take off, the pilot makes contact with the first in the series of airport controllers. Moving from the gate to the runway and into the air, your plane is "handed off" from one controller to another. As the plane moves beyond airport territory, you are transferred to the care of the controllers at en route centers. Like airport controllers, en route controllers stay in direct radio communication with the plane, use a radar map for tracking, and keep vigilant watch until they're ready to pass your aircraft along to another en route region. Finally, as your plane approaches the airspace of its destination airport, you are handed back to airport controllers. Your pilot is handed down the line, until the final ground controller rolls your plane home into its destination gate.

TIP Call the FAA office at your local airport. Many offer public tours or are simply interested in educating the public about air safety and can work something out. Ask for a program manager or public affairs officer, and let him know you're interested in touring the tower.

Inflight Sights, Sounds, and Vibrations

Passengers are often unnerved by the variety of unfamiliar sensations. Rarely do any of the flight attendants stop to explain what's going on during takeoff and landing—they're too busy checking exit rows, securing carry-ons, and fulfilling other FAA safety requirements. You won't hear from the pilots, either; according to the "sterile cockpit rule," no communication is allowed between the cockpit and the rest of the plane between zero and ten thousand feet, the area in which the plane is most likely to encounter turbulence.

After the last passengers have secured their carry-ons, and you're settled in your seat, you may hear **a range of thumps** that sound like they're coming from underneath your feet. These noises are from the loading of baggage, cargo, and food service units. When everything's aboard, the lower compartment doors will close with a **slam**.

As your plane pulls out from the gate and heads toward takeoff position, the cabin lights **flicker.** Interpreted by some passengers as a frightening omen, this flicker is in fact quite benign, marking the airplane's switchover from airport generators to its own electrical system. Next, you'll hear the **loud spooling** of the engines. The pilot is using the throttle to increase engine power. The cockpit is closed. This is not a sign of anything secretive going on, just FAA regulations, protecting the cockpit crew from any distractions.

Next, you will feel a **lurch** as the pilot releases the brakes.

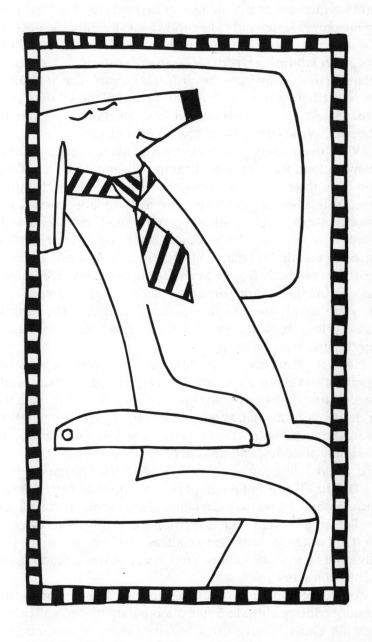

Whines and groans come from the hydraulic equipment that controls power steering and braking. Speed and acceleration increase as the plane moves down the runway. The plane moves faster and faster and faster still until the nose of the aircraft rises off the asphalt. A few final **bumps**, and then the main landing gear lifts. The steep, nose-up angle of the plane's climb away from the airport is normal. The dramatic-feeling **tilt** is a natural function of the plane's build and creates less noise above the neighborhoods near terminals (because planes don't fly as low for so long).

When the landing gear tucks up into the underbelly of the plane, a loud **ka thump, ka thump** will sound like it's coming from the floor under your seat. This is called "cleaning up." You'll hear a **grinding** noise as the plane extends its shock absorbers and pulls everything used for takeoff and landing inside, reducing resistance as the aircraft moves through the air. You may feel slightly light-headed, and notice that your body feels heavier during the ascent. Some passengers mistake these sensations for feelings of dread, but they are simply the effects of pulling up against the earth's gravity. Lean back and enjoy. This is a good time to settle in for daydreaming or sleep.

If you're sitting near the middle, you can see the flaps, slats, spoilers, and ailerons on the back of each wing **adjusting and readjusting**, helping to navigate the aircraft to cruising altitude. As your airplane continues to increase its speed, the wings begin to **flatten**. Less lift is necessary as you reach more desirable altitudes, and less curve means less drag.

If you're flying at night, you may notice that the main cabin lights **dim**. This is not a sign of power failure, but an FAA requirement. The relative darkness allows seatbelt warnings and other "message" lights, including exit-row designations, to stand out more brightly in contrast. Feel free to use the individual lamp switch above your head for work, reading, or a little company.

Your pilot may or may not get on the loudspeaker to announce cruising altitude. Some pilots are chatty and will point out the Grand Canyon, the Sonora Desert or the muddy Mississippi. Some pilots just fly the plane. If, at some point during your flight, you look out and register that this is not the way to your house, don't panic. There are many nonemergency reasons to reroute, like avoiding a thunderstorm or unexpected air traffic. Summon a flight attendant at any time for explanation.

The signs of descent are pretty clear. First, everything gets very **quiet**. The pilot is retarding the throttles. As the plane decelerates, you'll feel yourself **moving slightly forward** in your seat. The pilot will probably choose to coast for a while. This is a very natural illustration of the reason a plane will *not* fall immediately if its engines fail. Given some altitude to play with (and remember—we started out at around thirty-five thousand feet), even the largest commercial airplane can glide beautifully for about seventy miles. The aircraft's forward movement creates lift. The speed of descent keeps the plane aloft and controllable.

After a period of coasting, the noises change. "Stuff," as one commercial pilot put it, "begins to hang out." He was referring to landing gear, wing flaps, and all the accessories used during takeoff. These come back out with great **thumps** during the landing process, helping to slow and guide the plane. The throttle **roars** back up, holding the plane at the desired altitude for approach. There may be surprising **turbulence** (surprising to you, not to the pilot) as your aircraft moves down toward the runway; remember that warm air off the earth's surface creates uneven currents.

Your plane will touch down onto the runway with more or less **impact**, depending on the persisting air currents. Runway tarmac is sturdy stuff: it's made of asphalt layered over a foot and a half of concrete, cordoned with steel. If pressed, most planes could come to a complete halt in one-quarter of the available length, but the stop wouldn't be very comfortable for you or the landing gear. Commercial aircraft usually take a little over half the runway to land. The tires **spin shrilly** as they touch down on the runway, and flaps on top of the wing extend to deter lift and create resistance.

Solidly on the ground, the plane will continue to **brake**. As during takeoff, hydraulics **whine**. Your aircraft slows itself down, and turns in toward the gate.

Welcome.

·5·

If You're Still Having a Hard Time

If you've tried using guided imagery and understand how a plane stays in the air but still find yourself quaking at the thought of getting on a plane, consider the following options:

Desensitization

Start out by imagining an airport in your mind. At the same time give yourself messages to be calm and relaxed. When you can see an airport in your mind and still feel calm and relaxed, move in closer. See yourself going through the door of the airport, checking in at the reservation desk, going down the corridor to the gate, sitting in a seat at the gate, boarding the plane, etc. If at any point in this fantasy you become anxious, stop. Go back to the point that preceded your anxiety. When you are calm again, proceed, or stop the fantasy and try it again at a different time.

When you can go through the entire fantasy of going to the airport, boarding a plane, flying to a destination and deboarding the plane feeling calm and relaxed, it's time to try this out in reality. Take a trip to an airport. (You may want to take along a supportive friend.) The first time, you may want to just get close enough to view the airport from a distance. The next time actually go to the airport and walk in. On a third trip you may want to have a cup of tea at the airport restaurant. Take it slowly, and if at any point you become anxious, go back to whatever feels comfortable.

You may be able to arrange with an airline to actually board a plane and try sitting in one of the seats. Eventually, you'll be able to go to the airport, board the plane, and have a relaxed flight.

Therapy

Look for a counselor in your area who specializes in aerophobia. Your travel agent may be able to help you with this. In some areas of the U.S. you can call the licensing boards for social workers or psychologists. You might try looking in the yellow pages. You can always call a therapist and ask if she specializes in this, and if she doesn't, if she can recommend someone who does.

Feel free to ask questions over the phone about fees, experience with phobias, the specific approach used, and ask for an estimate of how many sessions would be necessary. If there is no one in your area who specializes in aerophobia, your next bet would be a therapist who specializes in anxiety disorders.

Fearful Flyer Programs

There are a variety of courses developed for fearful flyers. Sometimes they are offered by airlines (United, American, and U.S. Air all have them) and sometimes by community colleges. They vary in price. They offer the structure and support of a class and in some cases they take you on board a plane and show you around, which some people find helpful. Airline-sponsored programs usually include a "graduation flight" on a commercial airliner. The success rate is reputed to be high: 70 to 95 percent.

The Fearful Flyer's Resource Guide by Barry Elkus and Murray E. Tieger provides a listing of workbooks, video and audio tapes, individual and group therapy providers, and thirty-five national and regional seminars designed to treat the fear of flying. To order, send $13.95 plus $3.95 for handing to: Argonaut Entertainment, 455 Delta Avenue, Cincinnati, OH 45226 (513/871-2746).

II

TAKING CHARGE *of* YOUR OWN COMFORT

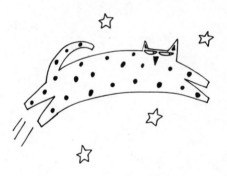

·6·

Schedule to Avoid Delays

You can start making your flight more comfortable the moment you book your tickets. To reduce logistical stress, take the following scheduling concerns into account.

Air Traffic Patterns

High air traffic volume slows things down. The busiest times above major airports are usually between 7:30 to 9:30 A.M. and 5:30 to 7:30 P.M. Monday mornings and Friday evenings tend to be particularly congested, as do the days at either end of holidays. There are other predictable high-volume periods as well, and these differ from airport to airport. Controllers manage daily flurries of activity, for example, when East Coast morning departures land in Denver, or flights from Asia reach San Francisco en masse.

The advantage of booking during "rush hour" is the subsequent ease of making connections. As part of the main wave coming in from the West Coast, you can take advantage of the long row of planes waiting to fly the next leg.

The disadvantage of booking during heavy use times is that one is more apt to encounter delay. If weather or other complications slow air traffic, your plane will have to wait at the end of a long queue.

Any travel office or ticket agent can let you know about general air traffic trends for the regions in which you're flying. When it's possible to travel during a less popular time and still get a good connection, do it.

TIP Always call the airline to check the departure time before you head for the airport. More and more schedules are changing at the last minute, and delays can happen at any time. If your flight has been bumped up or back, ask what the new gate appearance time is and prepare to meet it; if your flight has been canceled, you can rebook immediately.

We recommend using a travel agent, rather than an airline ticket agent, to buy tickets. There is no advantage to buying directly from the airlines. A travel agent will *not* cost you more. Travel agents do the footwork for you: They can cross-check pricing from airline to airline, issue boarding passes with greater flexibility, and automatically register frequent flyer miles once membership numbers are on file. They may even take last-minute reservations before special fares run out, giving you twenty-four additional hours to pay. Travel agents are generally more knowledgeable and customer-service oriented than their airline counterparts, and coordinate a wider variety of travel services, such as ground transportation and lodging.

TIP For any of the fourteen largest U.S. airlines, ask your ticket or travel agent for the "on-time arrival performance" of the flight you're considering. This information comes up on the agent's computer as a number between zero and nine. An eight indicates that the flight in question, during its last monthly reporting period, landed within fifteen minutes of scheduled arrival 80 to 89 percent of the time, a seven indicates punctuality between 70 and 79 percent, etc.

Crossing Time Zones

When crossing three time zones or more, we recommend you book a flying time—if at all possible—that helps your body adjust to the time change.

Flying west to east is generally more difficult for your internal clock. Therefore, try to plan a late afternoon or evening arrival. That leaves just enough time to get settled in, take a brisk walk, and eat dinner. This schedule makes it easier to sleep on local time.

Flying east to west is less taxing; an evening arrival is not crucial. The important thing is to stay active until local bedtime. See Chapter Twenty-two to learn how to reduce the impact of crossing time zones.

Flight Classification: Connecting, Nonstop, and Direct

The first transcontinental flights took a total of forty-nine hours—including something like twenty takeoffs and landings and two night stretches by train—to carry passengers from New York City to California. You'll never have to go through what they endured, but unless you're careful, you may end up touching down more often than you want to. Understanding the significance of flight classification will allow you to choose the schedule that best suits your needs.

Connecting is self-explanatory—the flight is scheduled to land and transfer passengers to another plane before reaching its final destination. The terms "nonstop" and "direct," however, are often confused.

Nonstop means what it says; your plane is going to fly from point A to point B without stopping. **Direct** flights stop between A and B, sometimes more than once. Passengers may not have to get off the plane, but they do have to sit and wait for new travelers and freight before continuing on.

If you're not in a hurry, the extra ground time is no big deal. If you are, unanticipated touchdowns are a frustrating waste. Know what you're in for. When time is of the essence, search out a nonstop. Confirm with your travel agent at the end of the conversation by asking, "These are nonstop flights, right?" Much to the annoyance of passengers, especially flyers who dread takeoffs and landings, nonstops are becoming less and less popular with the airlines. If scheduling the least possible number of stops is important to you, work with your travel agent to find the best schedule at a reasonable price.

The Official Airline Guides publishes several different *Pocket Flight Guides,* particularly useful for business and other frequent travelers, that lists arrival and departure times, number of stops en route, meals, and toll-free numbers for many airlines and hotels. A one-year subscription to the *North American Pocket Flight Guide* is about $90. Official Airline Guides, 2000 Clearwater Drive, Oak Brook, IL 60521 (800/DIAL-OAG). An on-line, electronic version is also available ($25 initial hookup, 17¢–47¢ per minute use fee). Many airlines publish system timetables for their own flights, available free of charge at airport ticket desks or by calling the appropriate reservations number.

If you're on a long haul, consider *purposefully* scheduling a direct or connecting flight that features a healthy layover. The extra time between flights can be used to stretch and walk around, which will elevate your spirits and reduce the consequences of jet lag.

Business travelers can treat the extra time like a stop by the office; they can fax, E-mail, or FedEx documents they've been working on, send messages or check in with the office on a phone with good reception. (See Chapter Twenty-one for additional suggestions.)

The ABCs of Seat Selection and Boarding Passes

Where you sit *does* make a difference. Whether you're traveling first class or scrambling first-come-first-served on a no-frills airline, you can increase the comfort and convenience of your flight by choosing a seat intelligently.

There are three different passenger classes: coach (economy), business, and first. Not all three, however, are offered on every flight. In general, short- to medium-length domestic flights sell coach and first-class seats, while the larger airplanes used for international flights offer all three.

Which Seat Is Best?

There is no "best" seat on the plane. Like everything else when you're traveling, good seating is a question of priorities. What matters most to you?

First Class vs. All the Rest

Flying first or business class can cost up to ten times the price of coach. Here are some essentials for understanding and evaluating the worth of the ticket to you.

The seats, though cushier, are not appreciably wider. The average width in economy is eighteen inches. Business boasts a slightly more generous twenty-one inches and first class twenty-two. Most of the extra money you pay shows up around your feet. Average *pitch*, the distance between your seatback and the upright seatback ahead of you, is more impressive: economy, thirty-one inches; business, forty inches; and first class, a calf-stretching sixty inches.

On most planes, a fully extended first- or business class seat goes almost all the way back and a footrest elevates the legs. One executive who flies regularly to Australia insists that "business class only" be specified in his compensation package. For him, this is the only way to guarantee enough sleep to do his job. The passenger in an empty coach section, however, may ultimately have the best option: while the armrests in first and business class usually don't go up, this traveler can push armrests out of the way, stretch out, and snooze on a completely flat surface. Working alongside a knowledgeable travel agent to schedule flights during off-times may reward you with more room than money can buy.

From linen tablecloths to Dior amenity kits, first class does communicate a certain aura, a sense of comfort and prestige. As a first-class passenger, you'll probably get heavy cutlery, real glass and porcelain, and a seatback viewing screen. Your part of the plane will be curtained or cordoned for quiet and "privacy." Some travelers even maintain that flight attendants are friendlier to business and first-class passengers, but we think that's a function of human nature and simple math: in coach, the same service is just spread more thinly.

Airlines insist that first-class and business meals cost between $25 and $60 per plate (as compared to $4–$7 in coach). First-class food *is* more artfully arranged, the menus are planned by renowned chefs and feature significantly better wine lists. Remember, however, that airline food is prepared hours in advance and reheated for passengers. No first-class meal will ever compete with a gourmet meal on the ground.

Perhaps the most alluring perk is the "executive lounge" available to business and first-class travelers. What amenities does any particular airline offer? Ask the reservations agent. Lounge services may include free local calls, bar snacks, espresso drinks, and international newspapers, as well as a host of slick business services—fax machines, modem ports, and private conference rooms. Are there other ways to access these facilities? Yes. See Chapter Twenty-one for information about purchasing membership.

Is flying "upper" class worth the money? Most frequent fly-ers say no, unless flying time is over three and a half hours. And then? Only if the advantages are worth it to you. There's no doubt it's cushier, but cush is relative.

Aisle, Window, or Middle?

On her computer screen, your agent can pull up a seating blueprint of the plane. This blueprint is a clear visual guide, like the layout used to sell seats at a concert. (You can access some of the same information—layout and facilities for different aircraft body types—in the back of an airline system timetable or OAG *Pocket Flight Guide* or *Travel Planner*.) Your agent can see the relative width of the plane, where the exit rows, smoking section, and lavatories are located, which seats are closest to diaper-changing or accessible lavatories, and which areas are getting full.

Aisle. Aisle seats are good for easy access to luggage stored overhead, multiple trips to the lavatories, and quick de-planing to make tight connections. They offer more leg room for tall people. An aisle seat is not a good place to sleep and leaves you prey to being jostled by anyone who walks by. Plan on moving aside to let seatmates out—more frequently if they're carrying their own bottled water.

In a wide-bodied plane, an aisle seat in the middle section may be preferable to an aisle on the side. If there are only four seats in the middle section, and two of these offer aisle access, only one passenger will be climbing over you to get to the lavatory. If you're scheduled on a wide-body with seven seats across the middle, however, an aisle seat in the center section is not such a great deal.

Window. The window seat, which enjoys the best reputa-tion, can feel either cozy or confining. It's good for sight-see-ing—if it's not over the wing—and offers more than the usual head support for night flights and napping. Getting out to go to the bathroom is an effort, but you shouldn't feel guilty about asking your seatmates to fold up their tray tables. The outside wall is chilly, so if you're planning to sleep, grab a blanket for insulation.

TIP If there's a land feature or something else you really want to see, figure out which side of the plane faces the view desired. If either side will work, take into account the position of the sun (at the appropriate time of day) to avoid bright glare.

Middle. Veteran flyers roll their eyes when they talk about the middle seat. There's almost no advantage, except being able to sit next to a companion or business associate.

TIP If you're traveling with a companion—or are a couple with an infant for whom you've not bought a ticket—reserve the window and aisle seats. You may score extra room because the middle will be the last to fill. If someone does take it, you can always endear yourself later by offering to switch.

TIP When traveling alone, request a single aisle or window seat in a row with another single who's done the same. Again, the middle is the last to fill so you may fly in luxurious semisolitude.

Forward or Aft?

For quick deplaning: Very strategic for tight connections. The front is where business travelers crouch, ready to run for a fax machine as soon as the plane lands. (In smaller airports without jetways, you may be deplaning from the rear.)

For less of a crowd: Head for the back. It's noisier and apt to put you close to the kitchen and lavatories, but sparsely populated.

For minimal noise: Sit as far forward as possible, avoiding the galley and lavatories.

For a good view of the movie: Individual preferences vary on the subject of ideal distance from the monitor. Beware that some seats have no view at all. Ask your travel agent to research monitor locations for any given flight.

For the smoothest ride: Book a seat over the wing. If you tend toward motion sickness, this is a great place to be. Caution: Sitting over the wing may prove disappointing to sight-seekers—there's nothing to watch but blue, blue sky.

For the most space: Try the bulkhead row. (The bulkhead is the wall between first or business class and the rest of the

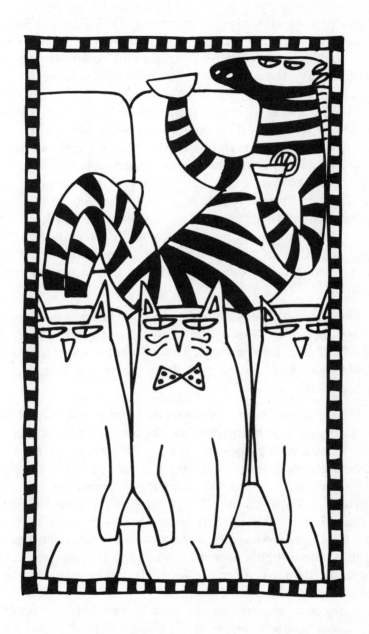

world). This row feels less cramped because you don't have to look at the back of anyone's head. Here, the armrests are nonnegotiable furniture; they house tray tables. And you'll have to store all carry-ons overhead. They'll be accessible during the main part of your flight but must be secured during takeoff and descent. Be aware that the bulkhead seats are often reserved by people with small children, or for unaccompanied minors.

The exit row is good for extra leg room, because the row *in front of it* will not recline. Avoid those seats. On planes with double exit rows, one right after the other, the first exit row's seatbacks will not recline (although armrests will lift). Remember that anyone sitting in an exit row must be prepared, and physically able, to help in the unlikely event of an emergency. No children. More and more airlines are refusing to assign these seats until they can personally screen passengers for suitability—at the gate. If additional leg room is important to you, consider arriving early at the gate to request exit-row seating.

For early service: If you're counting on airline food or beverage service and don't want to watch the entire plane sip their drinks while you wait (or you want to eat right away and get to sleep), sit near the front. Service almost always starts there.

If you are bothered by cigarette smoke: Ask where the smoking sections are before choosing a seat. On many flights, the first-class or business smoking rows are at the back of their sections. Nonsmokers sitting in the front of coach get a lung- full. Sit as far from the smoking sections as you can.

The U.S. Department of Transportation prohibits smoking on all flights within the fifty United States, Puerto Rico, and the U.S. Virgin Islands. This ban also covers domestic legs of international flights on both foreign and U.S. airlines. Any nonstop flight to or from Alaska or Hawaii, scheduled to last more than six hours, is exempt.

Carriers are required to provide a nonsmoking seat for every passenger who wants one—as long as those passengers meet airline check-in deadlines. The airline does not, however, have to seat you with your companion or give you your choice of aisle, window, or middle. If there are not enough nonsmoking seats to accommodate the nonsmokers who arrive at the gate on time, the airline must expand the size of its no-smoking section.

Most international flights offer at least one smoking section. Smoking is banned whenever the aircraft is on the ground, in galleys adjacent to no-smoking sections, and on all commercial aircraft seating less than thirty passengers. Ask your travel agent if there is a nonsmoking flight available on your route; some airlines offer them.

If you are tall: Again, go for leg room—the bulkhead, a window exit, a seat by the back door (on narrow-bodied planes), or an aisle.

If you are large: There are several good options. Tell the reservationist that you may need extra room, and if the flight isn't full you'd like to be placed next to an empty seat. In all but bulkhead seats, the middle armrest can be raised for additional space. You could also pay for two seats, or go first or business class. If the seatbelt is too restrictive, ask a flight attendant for a seatbelt extension; this is the piece held up during safety demonstrations.

If you are pregnant: For mobility, consider an aisle seat near the lavatory. For improved circulation, reserve a bulkhead seat so you can stretch your legs out and prop them up. Ask for an extension if you find your seatbelt too restrictive.

If you are disabled: Let the airline know what special requirements you may have. In situations where you'll need inflight assistance, take an aisle. Some of the newer planes have removable aisle-side armrests to make it easier to slide into the seat from a wheelchair. If you're traveling with a companion, think about aisle and middle, or try the aisle-and-window trick. See Appendix A for more information about accessibility, advance notice for wheelchair storage, companion requirements, and other related issues.

For the safest seat: Although you may hear a variety of opinions expressed on this subject, the leading authorities agree that all seats are equally safe.

When traveling with children: Specify the ages of children traveling with you when making reservations. Only one nonticketed infant or small child is allowed per row (there are four oxygen masks available to every row of three seats). Young people generally aren't permitted to take exit-row seating, either; FAA regulations require that exit-row passengers be willing and able to assist the crew in case of emergency.

The bulkhead is a great place for restless children; they can kick the wall in front of them, then play on the floor after the seatbelt sign flashes off. Do note, however, that bulkhead armrests don't move up and down; if your child likes to stretch out and rest on your lap, go for an alternative.

Changing Seats

If assigned a seat you don't want, talk to the desk agent as soon as you arrive at the gate. Ask him to hold your ticket until boarding, in case something comes up. Your physical ticket is an effective reminder. If no one calls your name, go back to the desk about twenty minutes before flight time and try again. When the prereserved seats are released, you'll be in line right behind the passengers holding VIP frequent flyer cards.

If you're already on board and want to switch seats, don't wait until after takeoff. (By then, someone else may have taken the seat you want.) Take a good look around as the time of departure nears. The moment before the aircraft door closes, make a move for your seat of choice. But remember: If you're on a direct flight, someone else may show up and claim that seat on the next leg.

TIP Rarely do animals travel in the cabin, but if you're severely allergic to animals you may want to check with a gate agent just before boarding to find out if there are carry-on canines or other pets aboard—and if they'll be sitting near you. A properly booked animal has the right to stay underneath the seat in front of its owner (in a carry-on kennel, of course). You can't make the owner or animal move but can plead with the gate agent to help you trade seats with someone down the aisle. If you feel strongly enough to want to change your ticket to another flight, put on your biggest smile: Whether or not this is allowed without a change fee is the decision of individual gate agents.

Boarding Passes

When you reserve tickets through a travel agent or airline reservations agent, you can save time and hassle by requesting a seat assignment and boarding pass.

Holding a boarding pass allows you to skip long lines at the front ticket desk. Your only check-in requirement is to report to the gate, which you must do at least fifteen minutes before scheduled departure time. (If you're planning to check luggage, a boarding pass gives you the option of checking your bags at the curb.) This extra time may be crucial if you're delayed in traffic, or convenient if you want to grab a magazine and a bite to eat.

TIP No-frills airlines offer seating on a first-come-first-served basis. Most start handing out their numbered boarding passes between ninety minutes and an hour before takeoff. There's only one way to beat being early. Pay a little extra—usually about $30—for a "business class reserved" seat. By reserving a seat in this manner, you can specify an area or type of seat on the plane and they'll hold it until takeoff.

While seating can be assigned at any time, your boarding pass will only be issued within thirty days of departure. This reduces the chance of a plane substitution after documentation is issued. If the new plane is of a different body style, for example, the substitution necessitates the reassignment of seating.

When you order tickets through an airline agent within thirty days of departure, boarding passes for both outgoing and return flights can be sent to you. Most airlines will use regular mail up to eight to ten days before the outgoing flight, and an overnight express service (charged to your credit card) when the timeline is tighter.

The only ways to get an advance boarding pass when you book within three days of flying time are: to buy your tickets at an airport desk, to buy in person from an airline office, or to work through a travel agent. If your return trip is scheduled for more than thirty days after initial departure, you won't be able to get a boarding pass for the return trip until you show up at the airport. If there is a dependable mailing address you can access while traveling, buy your tickets through a travel agent and arrange to have your return boarding passes sent there.

TIP Boarding pass or no, call ahead to confirm your flight. For domestic flights, the day before is adequate. When traveling internationally, call at least seventy-two hours in advance. Mounting pressure on the airlines to be cost-effective means tighter schedules and more last-minute changes.

·8·

Strategies for Eating Well

E ven if you think airline meals are nothing to write home about, count your blessings: the food of earlier flights was worse. One of the first commercial carriers, Transcontinental Air Transport, served a lunch of hard-boiled eggs and saltines with the belief that this bland fare reduced the possibility of airsickness. When they were able to lower the average airsickness rate to 75 percent, TAT believed they had reached a milestone in aviation history.

Today, most airlines contract out to large service kitchens for the provisioning, cooking, tray-laying, and foil-wrapping of their meals. It wouldn't be unusual to see United Airlines, American, and Northwest snack boxes all piled in the same kitchen; the cooks slice, sauté, and arrange meals for each according to the airline's respective recipe binders.

The amount of food consumed above thirty thousand feet is staggering. According to recent figures, in one month Delta fed a twenty-four-hour round of passengers departing from Atlanta in the following volume: 2,495 pounds of chicken, 2,698 pounds of lettuce, 19 gallons of olive oil, 519 pounds of butter, 18,532 dinner rolls, 920 pounds of coffee... and so on. The food is just as cosmopolitan as its high-flying consumers; butter wings its way eight hundred miles from Wisconsin, vegetables fly from California and Florida, the rolls travel seven hundred miles (frozen) from Chicago, and the apples 2,600 miles from the place apples grow best—Washington State.

TIP Make sure some of this food is on your flight before you count on eating it! Fewer and fewer flights offer full meal service. For coach passengers on board less than two hours, what once was a meal is now a snack, and what once was a snack has dwindled to one quick encounter with the beverage cart. On no-frills airlines the most you can hope for is a bag of honey-roasted peanuts. Going without food is no fun and can compound motion sickness problems. Check your tickets or call the airline before you fly.

Ordering Special Meals

The well-seasoned passenger is getting wiser: over four thousand passengers a day, on any given airline, order *special meals*. What makes a special meal so special? Special meals cater to the passengers—vegetarians, children, Hindus, diabetics, etc.—for whom the regular meal is not permissible, palatable, or preferable.

Anyone can order one. Today's special meal offerings on larger airlines read like a multicultural cookbook. United, for example, lists more than twenty special meals—and for any given category, you may get one of several alternative menus. Some are available during breakfast and brunch times, others lunch and dinner, and several all day long. Meal components have enough crossover that virtually any dietary restriction can be accommodated twenty-four hours a day. The following special meals are generally available:

Hindu Meal
Asian Meal
Cold Seafood Meal
Hot Seafood Meal
Kosher Meal
Fruit Meal
Pure Vegetarian Meal
Raw Vegetarian Meal
Lacto-Ovo Vegetarian Meal
Low-Calorie Meal
Low-Cholesterol/Low-Fat Meal
Low-Salt Meal
High-Fiber Meal
Diabetic Meal

Gluten-Free Meal
Baby Meal
Toddler's Meal
Child's Plate
Bland Meal

Though bland, this last meal option looks significantly better than TAT's: A typical offering might include grilled chicken breast, rice, broccoli, cottage cheese with a tomato, whole-wheat bread, and a slice of angel food cake.

A ticket or travel agent can tell you if food is being served on your flight, what the special meal options are, and describe a sample menu for each. When a special meal you'd like isn't available, let the airline know you believe it should be.

Unfortunately, a small percentage of meals never reach the passenger mouths they're supposed to feed. They are misrouted by computers, lost by loaders. While airlines work to perfect their systems, here are a few tried-and-true suggestions for making sure you get your goodies:

• **Order in advance.** Most airlines ask that you order meals a full twenty-four hours before boarding time (many quote less, but don't count on it). Record the name of the agent and the record locator number for your reservation.

• **Confirm before boarding.** When you check in for your flight, ask the attendant at the desk if your request is in the computer. If you arrive the recommended hour before your flight and a mistake has been made, there may still be time to load an extra meal for you.

• **Identify yourself to the galley attendant.** If you're scrupulously detail-oriented, check one last time with the galley attendant to make sure your meal's aboard. For fast, sure delivery, hand the attendant a piece of paper with your name, meal type, and seat number.

Brown Bagging

A market research executive who travels often around the United States, Europe, and Asia always packs her own meal.

She makes an event of it—drives down to a favorite specialty food deli, picks out marinated artichoke salad, a small container of good olives, a small loaf of freshly baked Italian bread. Wrapping everything securely in a sealable plastic bag, she stows her food at the top of a carry-on that fits under the seat. When she's hungry, or has been working on a report and is ready for diversion, she doesn't have to wait. And she doesn't have to gamble that when the meal cart reaches her, it will feature something that appeals.

We highly recommend this approach. Include a special treat. When you take your own food, you control when and what you eat. You know you'll be well nourished (if you want to be, that is). There's no feast-or-famine routine, no "I have to eat this entire tray of baked chicken and rice *now* or I won't get anything until tomorrow." Resist the temptation to take an airline meal just because the cookies look good. Airline meal service can last up to two hours. You'll be stuck balancing your own meal, and the airline's, on one tray table.

Pack so that your brown bag is easy to retrieve from your carry-on. Make sure the food itself is easy finger fare and requires no elaborate preparation onboard. Drain off excess liquids, like oil or salad dressing, before packing. Carry your own utensils. Plan to eat straight from your containers.

A convenient, portable tool, measuring about 2½ x 5½", the mini Traveler's Silverware Kit carrying case opens to reveal sturdy and artfully sized utensils: knife, fork, and spoon. Available from the Brookstone Company for about $10. See Appendix B for ordering information.

There are no microwaves aboard commercial aircraft and no standard ovens. Planes are fitted with convection-type ovens, form-fitted to hold the plastic serving trays; nothing else can be heated in them. There are no real refrigerators, either. Each plane has a "chiller" with cold air blowing through it. A passenger's request to store yogurt or bake a potato, therefore, will not be well received. Very hot water for instant soup, however, is available.

For greatest diplomacy, ask for hot water when the meal cart comes by. The ratio of passengers to flight attendant is usually much less favorable than the diner-to-waiter ratio in a busy restaurant. Flight attendants provide beverage and meal service *and* perform a variety of other duties.

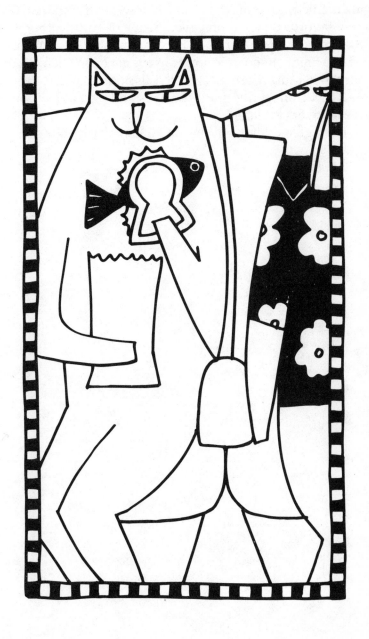

Especially if you have specific dietary needs (i.e., are diabetic, pregnant, or just plain like what you like), brown bagging is crucial to comfort. When you travel with children, take a few favorite snack foods, like raisins or fruit leather, and little boxes of juice. Although juice is available from the meal cart, the flight attendants won't always get to you before your children get fussy. Use plastic utensils and a Ziploc-type bag to protect from spilling. Plastic bags will also allow you to save leftovers for later.

A fresh green salad, a little good bread? Pack your own.

·9·

Manage Luggage Like an Expert

$\mathcal{G}$ ive careful thought to what will be most comfortable— and least stressful—for you. Want to check and forget it all? Travel toting little, and let the airlines do the rest. Need the ease of mind or scheduling convenience of keeping your belongings with you? Be ruthlessly spare in your packing and concentrate on carrying ease.

No matter what combination of luggage you choose, use carry-ons that are sturdy enough to be checked in a pinch; on the way home, you may want to hand carry your breakable gift or new painting instead.

Checking Your Luggage

Of the two million pieces of luggage handled by U.S. airlines every day, only ½ of 1 percent are lost, damaged, or don't arrive with their passenger. By checking luggage, the airlines do us quite a service: Checking luggage reduces fatigue. You don't have to slog checked luggage from gate to gate, juggle it during layovers, or cram it into crowded overhead compartments. Checking luggage also relieves mental stress; your checked bags become the airline's responsibility.

TIP Keep an eye on all check-in lines, disregarding the signs ("First Class," etc.) above them. Ticket agents will almost always let you check in when there's no one waiting in line.

"I'm far more likely to misplace my baggage between the restroom, gift shop, and Red Carpet Room," one executive emphasizes, "than the airlines are to lose it. And when I get off the plane, I'm going to have to use the bathroom and check in for a rental car anyway. What's the hurry?"

Airline limitations on the size and weight of checked luggage vary but generally allow two pieces—neither of which can weigh more than seventy pounds. If you need to travel with an abundance of goods, comparison-shop to find the airline with the largest allowance. Remember: Domestic and international limitations are different, even on the same airline. And while restrictions often go unenforced on domestic flights, international rules are followed more strictly.

If you're worried about losing your bags, check them early. If there is a mix-up, the airline will deliver your bags directly to you when they arrive. Arriving at the last minute, you may have to sign a "late baggage tag" before the ticket agent will check your luggage. This formality places the responsibility for your bags back in your hands. If your luggage is delayed, you've forfeited the handy doorstep delivery service. Be prepared to schlep back out to the terminal to fetch your bags.

If you have a boarding pass, you can save time and hassle by checking your bags at the curb. U.S. airport porters—known as "sky caps"—are airport employees; they are efficient, professional, and can be found on the sidewalks in front of most major terminals. Present your ticket and your bags about forty minutes before takeoff, and for the standard tip of one dollar per bag a sky cap will check and deliver them safely to the airline for loading. It's a good idea to make sure your flight has not been canceled or delayed by checking a monitor first (some airports have them at the curb).

If you don't have a boarding pass you'll have to go to the ticket counter. All you've gained by curb checking is freedom from carrying your heavy bags those last few yards.

▪ Remove tags from past trips. Make sure your luggage travels with you by asking for a translation of the three-letter code or codes—PDX, JFK, LAX, etc.—tagged on each piece, and checking to see that these codes are listed in sequence, with the *final* destination at the *top*.

▪ Tag both the outside and the inside of all your bags. On the inside, list your name, address and phone number. You may want to add the address or phone where you can be contacted in the days immediately following air travel. On the outside, list business information only, folding or clasping the tag discretely.

- To make your luggage more easily identifiable on the baggage carousel, consider tying a bright ribbon or piece of reflective tape to the handle.

- To keep checked bags as safe as possible from harm or intrusion: Lock main compartments whenever possible. Pilfering *does* occur. Remove shoulder straps and tuck them in a zippered side pocket.

- Make a quick list of the values for each item you've packed. Remember that airlines, like insurance companies, repay the *depreciated* worth of anything damaged or lost. Pack the list safely in your carry-on for use in the event of a baggage mishap.

Brookstone carries svelte, effective, and strong combination luggage locks that secure dual-zippered bags neatly. Set of three, $15. See Appendix B for ordering information.

Baggage beyond the two- or three-piece limit can be checked for an extra per-pound charge. Many airlines will send bikes and other bulky sports equipment as part of the allowed limit, *and* provide a carrying box. Ask individual airlines about their policies.

Airlines have the right to exempt themselves from liability for damage to "unorthodox" luggage—boxes, backpacks, fragile pieces, and the like. If you're checking one of these questionable items, a ticket agent may ask you to sign a waiver. (This releases the airline from responsibility for damage due to "normal wear and tear," but *not* damage resulting from their negligence.)

TIP Instead of using a cardboard box for one-way transport, use an old suitcase—for which the airline is liable—and donate it on the other end.

If you need to check extremely time-sensitive bags, like a box of presentation materials for an afternoon meeting, check them at the gate. Airlines discourage this, but it does work.

Make sure your bags will get through security, and that you can manage to carry or tote them all the way down to the gate. Tell the gate attendant you need to check your bags. You'll be able to watch airline personnel hand carry the items right down to the underbelly of your plane.

Which airlines handle baggage better? The Department of Transportation (DOT) requires the fourteen largest U.S. airlines to report the number of lost, damaged, delayed, or pilfered bags per thousand passengers. Find out how the airlines rank by calling the DOT (202/366-2220).

Traveling with Carry-ons

Smug in their self-sufficiency are those flyers who board with all their luggage in hand. They sail past ticket counter lines and baggage carousel crowds. These travelers get through customs before the crowd hits, grab a taxi or pick up the rental car with less competition. No luggage mix-up can touch them, even after switching planes to avoid delay; all clothing, amenities, and valuables are safe, secure, and in sight.

Typically, you are allowed one carry-on—two if the flight's not full. Length, width, and height combined can equal up to forty-five inches. The space under your seat, in the best of circumstances, will measure eight inches high, twelve inches wide, and twenty-three inches long. If your carry-on doesn't fit there, it will have to be stowed overhead. Room to maneuver outside official limits does exist but varies from carrier to carrier and flight to flight.

TIP Even if it seems like a hassle, ask about size restrictions for carry-ons when you book your tickets. Enforcement is becoming strict, especially during holidays and other periods of heavy traffic; some airlines have even installed "sizing boxes" at their gates into which your carry-on must fit.

Not everything you might want to take with you is counted as part of your carry-on allowance: a handbag, overcoat, umbrella, camera, reading material (within reason), infant bag, infant safety seat, and crutches can be portaged in addition to the basic one or two.

Oversized camera equipment—a video ensemble, for example—or an extra large purse, is counted as part of your allowance. So is a garment bag; permissible size is defined as the space equivalent of five suits. Want to take your cello? That's "cabin baggage." Pay 50 percent of the regular ticket price and strap it to a seat. (The one next to you.) It's possible to arrive early, endear yourself to a flight attendant, and stow large objects in the onboard closet, but don't count on it. Space priority for these closets is reserved for wheelchairs.

TIP The tri-fold type of garment bag fits under airplane seats most easily.

There's one final item in the long list of allowable carry-ons. For about $50, any passenger may use a secure, under-the-seat-fitting cage to carry their small dog, cat, or domestic bird. No guinea pigs. No snakes. And please note: Unlike your brown bag lunch, you may not unpack your companion during a flight.

If you fly with multiple carry-on items, make a habit of this exercise: Before boarding the plane, count the number of items with which you or your party is traveling. Say that number aloud: "We have five books, four bags, three coats, two umbrellas, and one cat." Repeat the phrase, checking to make sure it's still true, just before deplaning. Say it again before you board for the next leg, and so on. This combination of verbal and visual check-ins will reduce the chances of leaving your briefcase at the dried-fruit stand.

Include in your carry-on the basics for an unplanned overnight stay, just in case. Don't forget important phone numbers, prescription medication, contact lens paraphernalia, and extra glasses. Always keep your valuables—cash, jewelry, heirlooms, and important documents—with you. They're not covered by airline insurance.

Breakables should always be transported via carry-on. Wrap containers of liquids in plastic bags. Ziploc brand freezer bags work best—if the size is right—because of their thick walls and sealability. Pack a few extra; these plastic bags don't take up much space and will almost certainly come in handy down the road. Wrap your bagged items with softies you're planning to include: T-shirts, undergarments, pajamas.

Pack for accessibility. Place basic toilet articles (you never know when you're going to want to brush your teeth), books, or business papers—items you may want during a flight or layover—where you can get them without disturbing other bag contents. Use a side pocket, zippered top flap, whatever guarantees easy access.

No matter how you pack, keep one hand free to open doors, carry your water bottle, or call a taxi.

TIP Enhance your existing carry-on with a shoulder strap that is well padded and distributes weight effectively. Eagle Creek Outfitters offers a particularly deluxe model with a lifetime guarantee. The Ultimate Shoulder Strap retails for about $17. See Appendix B for ordering information.

Choosing Luggage for Comfort

Unless you're backpacking, luggage with wheels is almost always easier to manage than luggage without. Some options are more ergonomically satisfying than others.

The Rollaboard

Leading the pack is the Travelpro Rollaboard, replete with wheels, bountiful pockets, and a sturdy, retractable handle. Retired Northwest Airlines pilot Robert Plath started a revolution when he molded parts for the first model in his kitchen oven, adding the wheels from a Hoover vacuum cleaner. If you've been in an airport over the last three years, you're bound to have seen one. Rollaboards come in all shapes and sizes, including golf bags and computer cases; we recommend the original twenty-two-inch model, which can be checked or travel as a carry-on in an overhead compartment. It is extraordinarily roomy and comfortable to roll.

Other well-rated brands include Tumi, Skyway, Samsonite, and American Flyer. If you think this style of luggage might be your bag, test for:

A solid frame. The frames on these rolling wonders are made of either metal or plastic. While metal sounds like it's the heftier substance, beware—on some models, it's also more likely to bend. *Consumer Reports* found that luggage magnates like Samsonite and American Tourister are producing very sturdy plastic frames.

Durable bindings. If the space between the seam and binding is very slim, or the finish is bulky, don't count on that binding to hold. Where all seams are concerned, the closer the stitches the better. Leather-edge bindings, or those trimmed in nylon shell fabric or wide-woven tape, will hold up beautifully. Avoid plastic.

Good balance. Particularly crucial in a rolling bag, balance is a function of both the number of wheels and their location. When shopping for a bag, there's no substitute for weighting it down and wheeling around. Turn corners. Dodge travelers. Mime racing for the gate. (Luggage shopping can be fun.)

Tall handle. The main point here is that your handle needs to be tall enough for you to pull the bag along without stooping. In the airport, you'll be carrying things as well and you'll have to manage it all while covering long distances, quickly.

Attachment potential. The more items you can attach to your rolling bag, the better. Some manufacturers have planned ahead by including extra fasteners and clasps. The Travelpro Rollaboard features a solid metal hook for attachments, as well as a custom attachment method for other pieces of their own luggage. Elastic bungee cords may work but are less reliable. Look for a secure method of affixing extras, then try the balance test again.

Consult the most recent issues of *Consumer Reports* magazine (available in most public libraries) for a current review of specific models and brands. Investigate the preferences of frequent travelers you know. What does your travel agent use? Shop around. Luggage used to go on sale twice a year in most major department stores; today, you can comparison-shop any day of the year and find a variety of prices. Finally, look for a lengthy warranty—lifelong, if you can find it.

To locate a retail source for the Rollaboard, contact: Travelpro, 501 Fairway Drive, Deerfield Beach, FL 33441 (800/741-7471 or 305/426-5996).

Portable Luggage Carriers

If you fall in love with—or already possess—luggage that isn't comfortable to carry, consider using a luggage carrier.
Shaped like a miniature trucker's dolly but collapsible and

with bungee cords that hold items to the frame, "wheels" come in two basic sizes. The smaller type packs up most easily for checking or stowing away but still carries quite a lot: two suitcases, a large box, and a briefcase, according to one traveler. Wheels are also useful outside the airport—for moving boxes into a convention hall, for example.

TIP If you use wheels to transport carry-ons, don't feel like you have to fold them up at the gate counter. Roll down the jetway, all the way to the plane door, before stepping out of line briefly and dismantling your rig. Deplaning, you can unfold and load up those wheels as soon as you step on the jetway.

Shop carefully. Some brands of wheels are awkward, unbalanced, and consequently difficult to use as well as unpack, store, and repack on the aircraft. Look for wheels with:

Bungees that fit into a secure nesting groove at the top of the handle and are spaced sufficiently apart to accommodate wide loads.

An adequate bottom platform. Try out your luggage, and other intended loads, to make sure you're getting the right bottom width. For maximum flexibility, we recommend a platform that folds out, then opens like a book for additional support.

A high, secure, extendable handle. You shouldn't have to stoop over.

A design that folds into a small, slim package so you can check or stow the unit neatly.

Remin Kart-a-Bag of Joliet, Illinois, manufactures several lines of durable, cutting-edge wheels, all highly acclaimed by veteran travelers. For more information and a list of nearby retailers, call 815/723-1940. Remin does sell direct, but always at the "suggested retail price." Buy closer to home for a better deal. Other recommended brands include the Folding Hand Truck and the Travelite Luggage Cart, both of which are available from mail-order sources. See Appendix B.

Dealing with Damaged, Late, or Lost Luggage

When your bags are delayed, the problem is not often long-lived. Usually, the airline will deliver them to your doorstep within twenty-four hours—and sometimes the same afternoon. In the meantime, ask an airline representative for an "overnight kit" of toiletries. They may offer vouchers good in terminal stores or small amounts of cash for reasonable purchase of necessities. If they don't, but you believe they should, ask to speak with a manager.

TIP If lost or late bags interfere with the purpose of your trip, ask the airline to arrange for the rental of substitute sports equipment, formal wear, etc. If you request what you need for day one, believing your bags will arrive shortly, but by day two or three find they're still missing, don't hesitate to ask for rental of or compensation for additional items you may need.

When your bags are damaged during flight, the airline will pay for the injury to both bag and affected contents. If you checked pieces at your own risk, the airline is still responsible for damage due to mishandling or abuse. Examine your bags carefully when you pull them off the carousel. If you wait until you get home, it will be more difficult to make your case. If you have locked your luggage but see the lock was violated during flight, open your bags immediately and check the contents for theft or damage.

Filing a Claim

- Fill out a claim form *before* leaving the baggage area. Many airlines will not honor claims filed later unless the damage is such that it could not have been discovered immediately. (In this case, you usually have twenty-four hours to file.)

- Make sure the form you're filling out is a claim form and not just a report. If the airline insists on beginning with the report, go ahead and fill out the claim form as well even if you can't yet submit it.

- Describe the full extent of loss or damage to both bag and contents.

- Keep a copy of the paperwork, your baggage claim stubs and what's left of your ticket. You will need all of these, or photocopies of them, to prove your loss.

- Provide thorough contact information so the airlines can find you.

- Ask for the name of the agent who took your claim. Get a number for the on-site airline baggage services office—not just the corporate toll-free line—and maintain contact with the local office. Local personnel are much more likely to respond to your concerns.

- Don't exaggerate your claim; beyond obvious karmic concerns, the airline will reject your case the moment they sniff a fraud.

- If you are dissatisfied with the way your claim is handled or resolved, call or write the airline's customer service office with a well-documented complaint.

- You can also file a formal complaint against any U.S. carrier with the DOT if you feel the airline has not responded adequately. Send a letter and copies of all applicable correspondence to: Consumer Affairs Division, Room 10405, Office of Community and Consumer Affairs, Department of Transportation, 400 7th Street S.W., Washington, DC 20590 (202/366-2220). Be sure to note your daytime telephone number.

Airline Liability on Domestic Flights

The domestic U.S. liability limit for lost, damaged, or delayed checked baggage is $1,250 per passenger on all aircraft with more than sixty seats. This liability also applies to flights on smaller aircraft if they're listed on the same ticket with the big planes. This is the amount mandated by law that any airline has to pay—for *all* your baggage, no matter how large the actual loss.

Airline Liability on International Flights

Your baggage rights as an international passenger are guaranteed by one of several versions of the Warsaw Convention, a treaty dating back to the 1920s. The version most countries (including the U.S.) follow mandates a very modest checked-baggage liability limit of 250 French gold francs per kilo which translates—according to a U.S.-designated exchange rate—to $9.07 per pound. For carry-ons, the limit is $400 per passenger.

The airline must either record total checked baggage weight on your ticket, or assume each bag weighs seventy pounds. If the ticket agent doesn't note your baggage weight, make sure the fine print on the back of your ticket spells out the seventy-pound assumption. (The domestic leg of an international flight is covered as part of the international flight.)

Beyond Standard Airline Liability Limits

You may already have some insurance that covers baggage losses. Check your renter's or homeowner's insurance policy to see if luggage is covered. If you purchased your tickets by credit card, call cardholder services to investigate potential coverage there. If you want to buy additional insurance, ask your travel agent what he knows about extra coverage; some agents even sell insurance. It tends to be more expensive than other options, but if you've got something valuable to insure, it's worth looking into. In the event of a luggage problem, use any extra insurance to cover the difference between airline liability and the true value of your lost or damaged items.

Most carriers offer "excess valuation coverage," which increases the amount of compensation for which they are liable. Charges range from about fifty cents to two dollars per hundred dollars of additional coverage, with a common limit of five thousand dollars. Coverage usually excludes valuable antiques, jewelry, cash, camera equipment, computers, etc., but may cover some items the airline would otherwise insist you send at your own risk. Be sure you know what's covered, and what's not.

·10·

The Advantages of Arriving Early

Most airlines recommend arriving at least one hour in advance of departure (two hours for international flights). You probably scoff at this, considering the "extra" time excessive and mostly for the convenience of the airlines. If so, think again. Arriving early works to *your* advantage.

Being early keeps you safe. Airline passengers are seven times more likely to be involved in a car accident on the way to the airport than they are to experience any inflight emergency. Leave for the airport with plenty of time to spare, drive defensively, and secure parking without panic.

Being early prevents lost and delayed luggage—at least to the degree that it's preventable. We're willing to bet that most misrouted bags were checked at the last moment. When baggage loaders have to go running around after strays, mistakes can happen. Check your bags at the ticket desk *an hour* before departure, or *forty minutes* ahead at the curb.

Being early guarantees your rights. In the event of delay, overbooking, or cancellation, your rights as an air traveler will only be protected in the U.S. (and in many other countries) if you meet airline requirements for timely check-in. See Chapter Twenty.

Being early gets you grounded. Instead of trying to shave off as much airport time as you can, try on a new attitude. *Plan* to have "extra" time and enjoy it.

Use it to consciously slow down. Hurrying creates anxiety. Conversely, slowing down allows you to relax. Consider slowing down the minute you leave home. Drive leisurely to the airport. Once there, walk slowly, and slow your breathing. You may even want to slow your speech.

Indulge yourself with the extra time. Bring a book, a friend, a letter to write. Plan something fun and productive.

If you struggle with flight anxiety, this is a good time to do some deep breathing and establish the anchor points discussed in Chapter Three. Find a comfortable place to sit. Start with putting your feet flat on the floor. Feel yourself becoming calm. Let your favorite fantasy take you out of the airport. Listen to your taped instructions or soothing music.

By arriving early, you can avoid the stress that crops up with the unexpected or inconvenient: crowds, construction in the middle of the main terminal, a long line at security.

Being early may also get you: a better seat, onboard sooner, extra space, and a walking tour of the cockpit. Fifteen minutes before boarding is the time to take advantage of no-shows. We recommend you get to the gate even earlier. Winning tactics for changing your seat assignment are given in Chapter Seven.

When the desk agent announces preboarding, feel free. Let him know you feel you need a little extra time to get settled. If you're worried your carry-ons may not fit in the overhead compartment, you'll have extra time to find room, in the calm of a sparsely populated plane. If you're traveling with unusually unwieldy carry-ons, like paintings or musical instruments, there may be space in the plane's "flight closet" if your request is made early enough and no wheelchairs are aboard. Board as soon as possible, locate a kindly flight attendant and ingratiate yourself.

If you want to visit the cockpit before takeoff, tell the greeting flight attendant as soon as you board the plane. She'll let you get seated, then usher you forward to make introductions. The folks in the cockpit are usually friendly and flattered by your interest in their jobs. For an unusual experience, ask to hear the plane's "alert" sounds. Your pilots will show off their instruments, dials, lights, and buttons, as well as their slick view down the nose of the aircraft.

·11·

Navigate Security Checkpoints with Ease

While security checkpoints provide a necessary service, most travelers—especially those in a hurry—consider them a nuisance. Whether or not you're pressed for time, you may want to incorporate the following suggestions for increased ease of passage:

- When choosing between lines, look for one with more business travelers. You'll know them by their pressed suits, garment bags, and briefcases. The average business traveler knows the ropes, carries little with him, and wants to move *fast*. Holidaygoers and other flyers tend to have more shopping bags and wear more jewelry, which holds up traffic. They are less well versed in checkpoint restrictions and have more time to dither.

- Shed those items you think might set off the alarm *before* you walk through the metal detector doorway. This includes keys, coins, and heavy metal jewelry. Hand them to an attendant as you prepare to step through the doorway, turning quickly once through to recover them and move on your way.

- If it's too inconvenient to strip everything off, try cupping your hands over the earrings, bracelet, or belt buckle you think will set off the alarm. Your hands may be enough to shield offending items from the sensor, especially if you're not wearing much other metal. (If this doesn't work, you will have to de-accessorize and walk through again.)

- Lay bags and other carry-ons as flat as possible on the conveyor belt; if the person behind the TV monitor sees a jumbled image, he may want you to unpack or put your bag through again.

- Alert the attendant to any unusual items you anticipate will attract attention, including those that could resemble weapons. "There's a miniature antique silver violin from my grandmother in there." Satisfied by a reasonable explanation for the strange shape on the monitor, he's less likely to insist upon examining it. If you're really pressed for time, unpack the item ahead of time and ask for a hand inspection.

- If the alarm goes off, volunteer the explanation immediately: "It's my (gold ankle bracelet, iron belt buckle, steel-toe boots)." If the attendant knows the alarm was caused by an isolated object and has a partner with a scanning wand, he'll wave you along to her.

- One way to make sure you'll miss the flight is to joke about a hijacking or a bomb. Security officials will not only pull you out of line for a rigorous search, but you may also be charged with a federal offense.

The use of radiation in security screening makes some travelers nervous. Bear in mind that only those belongings placed on the conveyor belt scanner are subject to radiation. On the scale of radiation-producing machines and devices, airport security equipment (in all but the poorest countries) ranks at the very bottom. There is no appreciable residue left on belongings sent through the screening apparatus. This is true even when personnel freeze an object on their monitor. They are just taking a closer look at the image on the screen; no more radiation has been used than if the object had passed straight through.

The walk-through door is a metal detector that uses magnetic fields and emits no radiation. Some pacemakers may be sensitive to the magnetic properties; check with your doctor. There is no evidence that either the x-ray scanner or the metal detector is harmful to health except for those with pacemakers. But film and certain recording media can be damaged.

Film

Don't send film through the x-ray scanner if you can help it—especially film higher than 1000 ASA. The x-rays can mar film, creating unwanted lines or fog. The effects are cumulative, making this a larger issue if you have multiple security checkpoints to pass through. Be particularly vigilant in "developing" nations, where machines are less regulated and often emit higher levels of radiation than elsewhere.

If you're concerned about your film, unload your camera and send it through on the conveyor belt. Then hand your film to an attendant before entering the doorway. (You can hand it either around or through the doorway; the metal detector can't harm your film.) Ask the attendant to hand check your film. In some countries, a tip may be called for.

Lead bags, the most basic of which can be purchased for under $15 at a well-stocked camera store, are supposed to protect all film completely. Professional photographers claim, however, that security personnel often crank up the power in order to see through the lead bags; pros never allow their film to be x-rayed. (It *is* the job of security personnel to see what you're taking on the plane. Since the lead bag shows up as a blob on the monitor it's not unreasonable that they would try to get a better look.)

TIP Save time by packaging film in transparent film canisters. Scavenge these from a newspaper photo department, if you can't find them anywhere else. Seal the canisters in clear Ziploc bags; security personnel can inspect these thoroughly without opening each separate canister.

Computer Equipment

Some travelers worry about the effects of security equipment on their computer drives, disks, and cartridges. X-rays (used by the conveyor belt scanner) are harmless to computer equipment. The metal detector doorway, however, contains *magnetic* fields, which can corrupt computer paraphernalia, videos, and other recording mediums. Remember to send yours on the conveyor, or have them hand checked.

·12·

How to Cope with Changes in Air Pressure

Although your plane reaches a cruising altitude of about seven miles, at no point do you breathe the severely thin air of thirty-five thousand feet. As a human, you couldn't. The bar-headed goose, flying high over the snow-capped peaks of the Himalayas is the only animal who comes close.

The atmosphere inside the plane normalizes to the more tolerable equivalent of a high mountain top—between seven thousand and eight thousand feet—where you still encounter dramatically lower air pressure than most of us are used to. We experience the lower pressure and the changes in pressure during flight in a variety of ways.

Ear Pain and Popping

Air flows from the outside world into your ear and through your ear canal to touch the eardrum. Under normal circumstances, this air exerts atmospheric pressure against the outside surface of the eardrum. The other side is also in contact with air at atmospheric pressure, but that air sneaks in the back way, through the Eustachian tube, which forms a passageway between the eardrum and the back of your throat.

Each ear, then, has this flexible membrane that acts as a divider between outside and inside air. When the air pressure on both sides is equal, the eardrum is limber, free to vibrate when sound waves hit it. This vibration is "hearing." But when there's a rapid external pressure change, the air pressure on the inside can't adjust as quickly as that on the outside. The eardrum bulges painfully away from the side exerting the greatest force (but remember, it's flexible).

On the way up, as altitude increases and the pressure of the cabin drops, your eardrum bulges away from the higher pressure of the middle ear. Yawning brings outside air into the Eustachian tube, thereby mixing the air and equalizing air pressure. This frees the eardrum. The "pop" you experience is the twang of that stalwart little eardrum snapping back into place. Swallowing and chewing gum also work well.

Equalizing pressure on the way down is a bit more difficult. The outside air is increasing in pressure and you have to find a way to bring your middle ear up to speed. The best technique is called the Valsalva maneuver but be cautious about using this technique if you have a cold, or if your ears are very sensitive. Hold your nose, close your mouth—close your eyes, too, if that helps you forget how you look—and blow *gently*. Feel that eardrum spring back into shape? You've just increased the pressure in your middle ear.

These changes in pressure can be particularly painful when you travel with a cold. The fluid that collects in your inner and middle ear makes adjustment more difficult (it's easier to change the pressure of air than liquid). Use a decongestant one hour before takeoff and landing or a nasal spray immediately before takeoff and landing. But practice moderation: Decongestants and other medications will dry you out, causing other types of irritation. Vick's or eucalyptus oil, dabbed discretely under the nose, also helps to expand passages. Most physicians don't recommend flying with acute sinusitis or a middle-ear infection.

If you anticipate difficulty, use the hot-cup method. Flight attendants are trained to administer hot cups to passengers in need, but they do so only as a last-ditch effort, as it steals valuable time away from the required ascent and descent routine. You, however, can administer this treatment yourself.

- Take aboard the airplane a small thermos with hot water, two plastic or paper cups, and several squares of paper towel.

- Place a folded bit of paper towel, perhaps doubled or tripled, in the bottom of each cup.

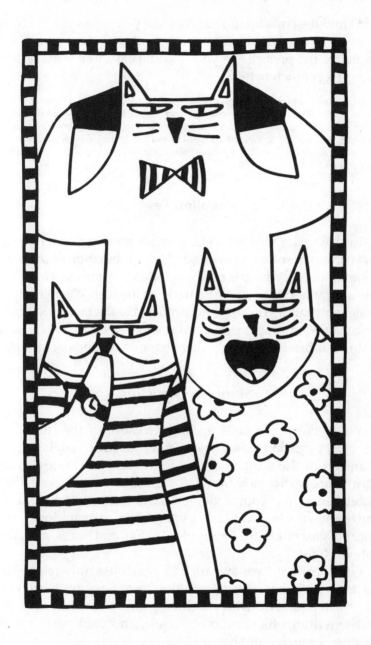

- Splash hot water (carefully) onto the layers of paper towel, just enough to wet the paper but *leaving no extra hot liquid.*

- Hold the cups up to your ears like you're having a private sort of phone conversation. The heat and steam will help equalize the pressure in your middle ear more quickly, and you'll feel much better.

Ear Ease, a smooth, plastic cuplike device patented by a pediatrician, achieves the same result. When you fill its outer chamber with hot water and hold the device over your ear, the heat provides relief within one to four minutes. The weight, warmth, and feel of Ear Ease are comforting and the device protects children from errant hot water drips nicely. Approximately $15, available from mail-order sources. See Appendix B.

Swollen Feet

Ever wonder why your dress shoes pinch so badly on the way from one plane to the next? The combination of pressure change and inactivity is hard on circulation and can cause uncomfortable swelling, particularly of the feet. Wear comfortable footgear. If you absolutely must take the tassel loafers or green suede pumps, stay in your shoes. Or slip a shoe horn into your briefcase to help them back on just before landing.

Sluggish Digestion

When the plane goes up and pressure in the cabin decreases, digestion slows down. You experience a relative expansion of the stuff in your tummy and intestines. Fizzy drinks are particularly troublesome and can make the seatbelt stretched across your abdomen quite uncomfortable. Minimize the effects of altitude by avoiding carbonation. Steer clear of gaseous foods like apples, melon, and beans, and simply eat light.

One frequent flyer swears by vegetable sandwiches. His fare never changes: fresh tomatoes, sprouts, spinach, a favorite mustard and fresh bread. Other good options include light carbohydrates like crackers, bagels, and cold pasta salad. Grapes, oranges, and bananas also go down well.

Scheduling Dental Work

When air pressure changes, the air or moisture left sealed in the space behind dental work can cause pain or loosening of a filling, cap, etc. The resultant toothache has a name: aerodontalgia. Consult your dentist or doctor before making travel plans close to dental work or oral surgery.

Attention, Divers!

Obey the rule: don't dive and fly. After a total bottom time of two hours, wait another twelve before flying. After more than two hours underwater, wait twenty-four. The body cannot tolerate the extreme changes in pressure caused by going from underwater to high altitude in a short period of time. Violation brings serious consequences, putting the diver at risk of painful and dangerous nitrogen bends. Plan your island itinerary carefully, and reschedule your flight if you find yourself in a squeeze. Contact a certified scuba instructor if you have questions.

·13·

The Truth about the Air up There

Aircraft air has received a lot of dubious press, fueling passenger concern about inadequate oxygen levels and the "sick building syndrome." The situation is not as grim as it sounds. Uncomfortable, sometimes, but no more threatening to your health than inhaling at a suburban shopping mall or a crowded party. The real culprit is the extraordinarily dry air of higher altitudes, which causes a degree of dehydration more severe than most travelers realize.

Breathing in a Crowded Space

Aircraft ventilation systems, which regulate circulation and the ratio of fresh air to refiltered, vary with each aircraft model. They maintain maximum comfort for passengers at reasonable cost and optimal energy efficiency. These systems work in one of two ways.

Some planes, like the Boeing 727, pull in 100 percent fresh air from outside the aircraft. Cold air—about 65° Fahrenheit at thirty-five thousand feet—comes in through the plane's jet engine compressors, where it heats to about 400°. A portion of this air is cooled to more comfortable temperatures by the plane's air-conditioning units and heat exchangers, which level the temperature by adding more chilly outside air.

Newer models, like the Boeing 767, combine fresh outside air with filtered, recirculated air. All cabin air is replaced with a mixture of fresh and filtered air twenty to thirty times per hour. Recirculation systems discard approximately one-half of used cabin air, while using fans to draw the other half through special filters. Standard home and office types are used in combination with the type used in hospital settings. A recent study by Consolidated Safety Services, Inc., at the request of the Air Transport Association, concluded that biological contaminants aboard these aircraft are low, especially for a confined space. Flying doesn't increase your risk of infection more than any situation in which strangers sit together—and maybe less.

So why do airplane passengers feel so awful?

What the experts have discovered is that when humans spend prolonged periods of time in an environment with high levels of carbon dioxide (CO_2), they often suffer flulike symptoms; office workers with sick building syndrome report overall sluggishness, sore throats and coughing, dry or watery eyes, and headaches. The longer a person is "exposed," the more extreme his symptoms may be.

Studies of "sick" environments, however, show no single bug or microbe in unusual abundance. Carbon dioxide seems to be the uncomfortable, but ultimately innocuous, culprit.

In the cabin of an aircraft, passengers breathe levels of CO_2 comparable to that of anyone who spends time in an enclosed, well-populated space. Humans breathe about five thousand gallons of air each day, at an average rate of something like twelve inhalations per minute. On an average cool, clear day, the air you inhale is made up of 21 percent oxygen and less than 1 percent CO_2. (The rest is nitrogen.) On the exhale, you expel air measuring 16 percent oxygen and 4 percent CO_2. The increase in CO_2 concentration aboard an airplane is a natural consequence of normal breathing—in limited space and for an extended period of time.

Here's the good news: Typical sick building syndrome symptoms begin to diminish within minutes of quitting a CO_2-ridden space and are usually completely gone after several hours. There is no indication that even the most frequent of flyers experience any long-term effects. Your upper respiratory tract, while sensitive, is also extremely forgiving.

People do seem to come down with colds frequently after flying, but there is no evidence that this has anything to do with undue air contamination aboard the aircraft. It is more likely that post-travel illnesses result from the stress of air travel itself, *particularly the effects of dehydration on the body,* which taxes the immune system.

So there's too much CO_2 up there. What can you do to feel better? Relax and breathe deeply, exercising the fullest possible lung capacity. Take advantage of stops and layovers: Get off the plane to stretch, walk, and breathe. Try to get outside when there's time. If you're asthmatic, fly with your inhaler handy.

Spending the extra money for business or first-class tickets buys more oxygen; the average coach passenger gets about seven cubic feet of fresh air per minute, while first class breathes in fifty. (Both sections of the plane receive the same amount of air, but in first class, fewer people share it.)

Finally, after you reach your destination, handle that upper respiratory tract with care. Take a steaming hot shower. Steer clear of smoky clubs and restaurants. And breathe, breathe, breathe.

TIP If the air on your plane feels stuffy, ask the flight attendant to request that the cockpit increase ventilation. Ask specifically for "full utilization of air."

TIP At press time, *Consumer Reports Magazine* rated air aboard the Boeing 757 as the stalest, while air aboard the Boeing 747-400 was the freshest. With the evolution of plane design, this information is apt to change continually; to keep abreast of the latest findings, watch sources such as *Consumer Reports* and *Condé Nast Traveler.* You can always ask your travel agent to formulate an itinerary based on your plane-style preferences and hope no changes occur before takeoff.

Breathing Desert Air

Severely dry air is the greatest enemy of the air traveler. The most desiccated desert regions on earth have a relative humidity level of 20–25 percent; airplane air measures only 5–10 percent. The cold, fresh air pulled in at thirty-five thousand feet is drier than dry, but airlines don't humidify because they don't want the extra weight, added expense, or risk of mold growth. So dehydration continues to make travelers lethargic, light-headed, and irritable. Skin becomes scaly, your mouth gets dry. Eyes burn, headaches rage, your hair even goes limp.

Dehydration is one of the main contributors to the ritual cold many travelers suffer after flying. It is recommended that adults drink eight cups of water a day. On a plane, you lose at least eight ounces of water—one of those cups—by evaporation from your skin *every hour*. Lack of adequate moisture places stress on the body, reducing mucus production and lowering the immune system. When your internal humidity level drops, your body becomes fair game for a vast assortment of aggressive microbes.

Follow these suggestions to stay well moisturized, and a great deal more comfortable, on your next high-altitude trip.

▪ **Drink lots of water.** Starting several days before your trip, pound those liquids. When it's time to fly, take your own bottled water aboard. You can buy it in the airport if you forget. The plain water supply aboard the aircraft isn't regulated for purity and, on longer flights, may dwindle to drought. So take your own, and don't be shy. Carry the biggest bottle you can muster.

▪ **Avoid alcohol.** It is a diuretic and will further dehydrate your body. (It also increases your chances of getting motion sick by interfering with the coordination between vision and movement.) If you do drink alcohol, go light: Due to the altitude, one drink in the air will hit you like two on the ground. Be aware that the histamines in wine can contribute to sinus congestion. If you do drink wine, bypass highly acidic whites and tannic reds. Their astringency only exaggerates the problem. A pinot or chardonnay is your best bet.

▪ **Avoid caffeine.** It also acts as a diuretic. Caffeine is found in coffee, tea, many carbonated beverages, and some over-the-counter medications. If you already have a caffeine habit going, don't abstain to the point of withdrawal; avoid nasty headaches by ingesting minimal amounts and at least eight ounces of *extra* water per caffeinated beverage.

▪ **Watch out for salts and sugars.** Whether or not you pack your own picnic, plan to eat foods low in salt and sugar. This helps your body retain the most moisture.

- **Pack travel-size moisturizers.** The condition of your skin is a good reflection of what's happening inside. Use of moisturizers won't rehydrate your body but will soothe skin irritation and make you feel better. Tuck lip balm and a general moisturizer into your carry-on.

Some frequent flyers are religious about hydrating eye creams, which are purported to reduce puffiness and moisturize the tender skin around your eyes. But topping the list of skin care aids is one recommended vigorously by flight attendants: a spritzer that mists refreshing, moisturizing ingredients over the face and body. The most refreshing spritzers are astringent, nonoily, and stimulating to the skin.

Garden Botanika, a natural products company, makes one with a clean, cucumber-like scent that appeals to both men and women. An eight ounce bottle retails for about $8.50 (800/968-7842 or 206/881-9603). Another brand that comes highly recommended for both hair and skin is Focus21 International's Seaplasma. You can call them to order or pinpoint a retail source (800/832-2887 in the U.S., Canada, and Mexico, or 619/727-6626).

- **Use familiar scents.** Although this tip doesn't specifically address hydration, incorporating a familiar, soothing or clean-feeling scent into your moisturizing efforts will increase general well-being. Humans are extremely sensitive to smell. Researchers have found that the smell of vanilla lessens anxiety. Lavender relaxes. Rosemary refreshes. The incidental waft of a favorite will make you feel cared for.

- **If you have sensitive eyes, use artificial tears. If you wear contacts, take them out.** The dryness of the cabin is especially hard on eyes. Consider removing your contacts in favor of glasses, particularly if you're on a long flight or plan to sleep. Regardless, it's a good idea to keep a small dropper of saline handy.

- **Take a hot bath or shower.** As soon as you can, steam away the dryness of the plane with a wet sauna or good soak. You'll feel energized and ready to go.

- **Keep drinking water.** During the days following your arrival, make sure you continue to drink extra water. The effects of dehydration tend to linger, so just keep guzzling.

We cannot overemphasize the importance of adequate hydration. You may think you're taking in lots of liquids when you fly, but we guarantee that if you drink even more you'll have a vastly better flight experience. Drink water. Then drink more water.

There are some high-tech alternatives. Passengers on Japan Airlines get their own gadget to try—the company's exclusive paper Honeycomb Mask, reportedly very effective. HumidiFlyer's $21 mask, however, is available to anyone. The whole apparatus fits over nose and mouth, making every wearer look like the same species of large insect. Inventor and former flight attendant Paul Aberhart came up with the design after suffering chronic sinus problems from dehydration. Aberhart claims that wearing his mask and filter contraption during flight will conserve about 86 percent of your body's own moisture. We've tried it, and we're tempted to believe him. Even strapping on the HumidiFlyer for a few hours after the meal service makes a big difference. The HumidiFlyer also helps to filter out cigarette smoke and offers a convenient medium for self-aromatherapy. Simply place a drop of your favorite essential oil in the filter of the mask.

For more information about the HumidiFlyer, contact: HumidiFlyer Technologies, P.O. Box 168, Neutral Bay, NSW 2089 Australia (02/953-9080; fax: 02/953-9080).

Coping with Smoking

Unfortunately, there are few clean-air options for nonsmokers on international flights or domestic flights outside the U.S. Because airplane air is recirculated and all passengers ride along in the same enclosed space, you're bound to come in contact with some amount of secondhand smoke. Your best bet is to secure a nonsmoking flight; ask your travel agent to investigate the possibilities thoroughly. If there are no nonsmoking flights on your route, at least choose an airline that has the lowest proportion of smoking clientele. Use your own experience with smoking habits in different countries, or ask your travel agent to compare the percent of seats designated for smokers from airline to airline.

Choose your seat to maximize your access to fresh air; it does make a difference. (See Chapter Seven for recommendations and the DOT's rules governing U.S. carriers.)

If secondhand smoke is a concern, consider using a disposable nose-and-mouth mask. Surgical masks are available from medical supply stores and some pharmacies. Even the white fiber kind found in hardware stores will significantly cut down on the amount of particulate matter you inhale. You may also be able to find the gray-tinted variety; the color is less obtrusive than white and doesn't tend to alarm other passengers. A military surplus store can outfit you with a gas mask to filter air more completely—if you're willing to wear the contraption.

In countries where cabins are sprayed with insecticide upon arrival, a mask provides some measure of protection.

Managing Volatile Temperatures

The temperature aboard airplanes tends to fluctuate from one extreme to the other. Running the plane's air-conditioning system uses a great deal of energy, so crews try to cool down the aircraft with airport units while they're hooked up at the gate. Once airborne, they are reticent to use the plane's own air conditioning. On a fully booked flight, things get hot. (The thermostat is in the cockpit. Kind of like letting a neighbor control *your* furnace from *their* living room, there's no guarantee the cockpit will get it right.)

The best way to fly at a comfortable temperature is to take control of your own microclimate.

▪ **Layer.** Be prepared for a range of temperatures, dress in layers, and take a few extra. A light shirt, simple cardigan or jacket, and a heavier sweater or overcoat should see you through almost anything. Warm socks, even if you're wearing dress shoes or nylons, are handy for slipping on at altitude. If you tend to be chilly, avoid the exit-row window seat. It's the coldest seat on the plane.

▪ **Ask for a blanket.** If you forget your layers, need another, or just want the feeling of being all tucked in, grab an airline blanket from the overhead compartment. There are enough for everyone, so if you can't find one, ask. A flight attendant will pull a couple from his secret stash.

▪ **Take full advantage of your air nozzle.** If you're too hot, reach up to the ceiling panel and direct the plastic cone right at your face. Twist it open to the left for the fullest effect. If you're cold, twist your cone to the right and shut it off. If your seatmate isn't paying attention, twist hers off, too.

▪ **Be vocal.** The copilot doesn't know it's 103° in the cabin until somebody tells her. You can summon a flight attendant and ask if he will please, please tell the copilot that at least one passenger is so hot he's about to take his clothes off—all of them. Would it be possible to turn that air conditioner up a teeny bit? This may or may not make a difference, but it is certainly worth a try.

·14·

Avoid Backaches

Have you ever disembarked feeling tired and sore? The aches could be from slogging suitcases or from the stress of the posture your body maintained during flight.

Our bodies weren't meant to sit, but deep breathing, good posture, and consistent, subtle stretching will help the muscles and organs cope with cramped cabin quarters. Knowledgeable positioning of the head, neck, legs, and back makes a tremendous difference in the way you feel after flying. And there's a bonus: Amid the stress and bustle of travel, this increased body awareness can be meditative and relaxing.

Posture

When we sit, especially in the seat of an airplane, we tend to lean forward. The back, shoulders, and neck crunch forward, while the head tilts slightly back to compensate. The key to comfortable sitting is to avoid this position.

Breathing

It's tempting, and typical, to breathe with the upper part of the chest while sitting, but abdominal breathing is crucial to avoiding strain and encouraging relaxation. Here are some things to focus on:

▪ Place your hands on your stomach. **Breathe into your stomach** so it pouches out. If it goes in when you inhale, you're breathing from the chest. You may want to put a hand on your chest as a backup; the chest shouldn't move at all.

- While maintaining good, natural abdominal breathing, **concentrate on bringing air in through your nose.** Rest your tongue on the roof of your mouth. This trick activates an automatic reflex that will help align the muscles in your neck.

If you've got a cold, hay fever, or are mildly congested, breathe through the nose anyway. Unless you're totally blocked up with something like bronchitis, the tongue-and-nose breathing trick stimulates an adrenaline surge that should clear you right up. If it doesn't happen within a minute or two, back off. Don't wait until you turn blue in the face.

- *Don't work too hard.* Some people try so hard to breathe correctly that they take themselves right over the top and get too much oxygen. This is called hyperventilating, and you'll know if you're doing it by the mild dizziness you feel. Don't get anxious; just reach for a (clean) airsickness bag and breathe in and out of the bag for extra CO_2.

Upper Body

We're all told to sit up straight, stand up straight. This feels good for a minute or two, then we're ready to give it up. Why? We're working too hard. The way to sit upright with the least strain is to concentrate on the sternum, or front of your rib cage. The trick is to do so without contracting the back muscles. As you begin to correct this posture, everything else will start to come together.

- **Don't tighten your shoulders.** Right now, sitting just where you are, put a hand on your stomach and take an abdominal breath. Your shoulders will drop and relax. Let them stay there.

- **Notice the rhythm of your own breathing.** Prepare to incorporate the next element in time with it.

- **As you breathe out, lift the sternum.** Everyone tries to do this while breathing in, which consequently tightens the back muscles. Your back muscles are meant to be used for power activities but not to stay contracted. To sit upright, you want to use deeper sustaining muscles. Communicating with these deeper muscles however, is difficult. That's why the breathing cues are so useful. Stay natural. Don't use your back muscles or bring your shoulder blades together.

Moving through the breathing sequence will take all of thirty seconds. Now is a good time to try a few shoulder circles:

▪ **Move your shoulders forward and around, then backwards** for more circles, maintaining your abdominal breathing. Have fun. Move the left shoulder forward and the right back. See if you can get them rotating in opposite directions.

The breathing routine—minus the shoulder circles and with your seat all the way back—is the perfect preparation for daydreaming, meditation, or sleep.

TIP Keep your seat straight up when you're active—reading, writing, or typing on your laptop. Use the tray table. The increased height is much better for your neck and back than using a laptop as its name implies. When you're reading, the tray table keeps elbows up and shoulders relaxed.

Bear in mind that our bodies weren't meant to stay in one position too long, even if that position is the "correct" one. Avoid holding the head-down position for more than ten minutes at a stretch. Even if it's just to look up from your laptop or the magazine on your tray table, take fifteen seconds to lift your head and look around. On longer flights, take slightly longer breaks.

Low Back

▪ **Sit with your feet flat,** no tiptoe action. Your knees should extend at an angle of ninety degrees from your trunk. Place a carry-on bag under your feet to bring your legs to this angle if you need to.

▪ If you've never had problems with your lower back, **keep your bottom smack up against the seatback** and you should be fine.

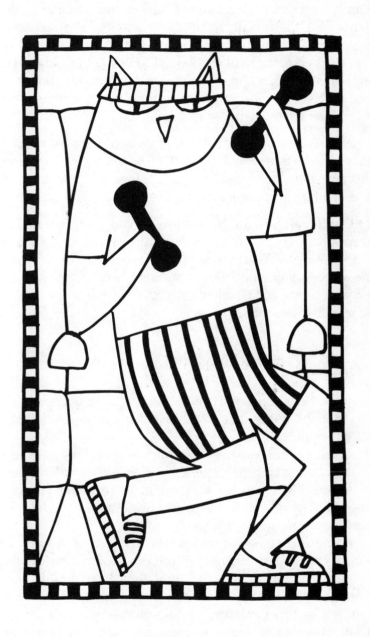

• **Use lumbar support** if you have back problems. The airline pillows and detachable headrests are the perfect size. Handy alternatives include a T-shirt or thin sweater, rolled tightly. For placement, scoot all the way back in your seat, then put the pillow or roll in behind you as low as it will go. Travelers commonly place their pillows a bit too high. The support should end up about the level of your hipbones. But don't force it: If your new back support feels too tight or too big, adjust the tool—not your body.

• **Avoid crossing your legs for prolonged periods,** particularly if you've had back pain. It's fine to look debonair for short intervals, but crossing your legs for more than five minutes at a time puts strain on your back. You'll feel it.

• **Don't maintain a rigid posture.** If you do have a history of back pain, try to sit no more than twenty minutes at a time. But if your plane is camped out at the end of a runway and the seatbelt sign stays lit for an hour, don't panic. Get up when you can, and in the meantime, do a few of the isometric exercises described below.

Stretching and Circulation

Our bodies are meant to move. During long periods of sitting you will notice that ankles swell and joints get tight; inactivity makes us stiff.

During a flight, especially a long one, *stay active*—even if your movements are just little shifts in the seat. Don't feel self-conscious. Get up to walk somewhere whenever you can. And when you're settled in working, eating, or reading, repeat a few simple isometrics.

Isometric exercises, movements that flex and contract muscles without utilizing their full range of motion, act like "muscle pumps" to activate circulation. Incidentally, these motions also alleviate cramping. When you're distressed by a muscle cramp, contracting a muscle that moves in the opposite direction triggers a reflex to relax the initial offender. A cramp in the calf, for example, can be loosened by contracting the shin muscle—flexing the foot.

- **Hamstrings and thighs.** Hook your feet under the seat in front of you. Contract the thigh muscles and stretch the muscles running down the back of your leg by trying to straighten each leg up against the seat bottom. Try alternating left, right, and both at the same time. Relax, then repeat. Try not to kick; there's someone sitting right on top of your workout studio.

- **Lower legs.** Again, hook your feet under the seat in front. This time, try to pull your toes back toward your head. Alternate left, right, and then flex both at the same time. Relax, then repeat.

- **Hands.** You can give your own hands a brief massage. Push tightness through the inside of the palms and out the ends of your fingers. Squeeze the muscular place between your thumb and index finger. Place the tips of your fingers together like a spire and arch them against one another.

TIP Many airlines now offer a video or audio stretching routine; check the airline magazine. British Airways, for example, offers a one-hour "Well-being Programme" that features soothing music, mild stretches, and relaxation techniques.

If you're taking in enough liquid, you'll need to visit the lavatory with frequency. One quarter of all passengers crawl over their aisle-mates to get to the bathroom every hour. Join them. Both the hydration and the walk are good for you. Plan to get up and move around or go through the stretches detailed above every hour you're in the air. If you sleep, stretch before settling in and again after waking.

No one can permanently change their posture in one plane trip or even a solid week of physical therapy. For maximum effectiveness on the plane, these techniques need to be practiced in the larger context of your life. At home, in the office, over an intimate dinner: Breathe, open your sternum, and sit relaxed with your feet flat on the floor. Every once in a while, get up to change the music. Practice sitting in a relaxed position, and you'll feel better at the end of your trip.

·15·

Escape Noise

The high noise level aboard a plane adds significantly to discomfort and fatigue. Everyone hears it but most passengers are not aware of the toll it exacts.

Do the extra decibels cause damage? The jury's still out. While the Air Transport Association of America asserts that cabin decibels measure "well below dangerous levels," other sources report that the inflight levels are close to 96 decibels (dB). Prolonged exposure to 100 dB can cause permanent hearing damage. The rustle of leaves is equal to 10 dB, and a normal conversation is 60 dB. Shouting clocks in at about 90 dB, and a loud rock concert measures 120 dB.

Scientists have discovered that when under stress, people perceive noises as louder than they actually are. The greater the stress, the louder they seem. If you struggle with fear of flying, you may feel particularly assaulted by noise in the air. Try giving yourself more quiet on your next flight. Travelers who use earplugs or headphones, even just while sleeping, report feeling *much* more rested and less worn by their experience in the air.

Earplugs

There are two basic types of earplugs: wax and foam. The wax plugs are effective and easy to use but kind of messy. It's embarrassing to walk through the terminal with a misshapen glob of earplug in your hair.

The more popular foam type looks like a pellet. Twist it to slightly compress the foam and insert the plug into your ear, where it quickly expands to fill up the available space. Unlike wax plugs, these can be washed up to ten times. Both wax and foam earplugs can be bought in drugstores, travel stores, and through mail-order sources. See Appendix B.

Some airlines provide plugs for passengers; it doesn't hurt to ask. If you find yourself without earplugs, at least use airplane headphones—volume off—when they're provided.

TIP For maximum soundproofing, look for earplugs with a rating of 26 dB or better (a foam pair rated 29 dB is the best option we've seen).

Headphones

One flyer felt that after using earplugs for a time, his ears were actually working harder to get at outside noise. They seemed to be reaching for sound *around* the plugs, and the plugs stopped being enough. Wanting to give those stimulation-seeking eardrums something to work with, but preferring to maintain an insulated environment, the man started flying with his portable tape player and found that he much preferred headphones to earplugs. Experiment to see which works better for you.

There is also a new type of headphone called the Noise Buster that purportedly reduces noise by emitting reverse sound waves to cancel out general, low-frequency sounds. Overall reports on the Noise Buster's effectiveness are mixed; it retails for about $150 and is available through many mail-order sources. See Appendix B.

·16·

Sleep Soundly

For many travelers, the ability to sleep is what determines the success of a flight. Particularly on overseas flights and transcontinental red-eyes, staring fitfully hour after hour at the seatback in front of you is frustrating. It would be so much nicer to drift off and wake refreshed, ready to jump into that business meeting or undulating surf. For a good night's sleep, follow the suggestions below.

Getting Comfortable

• **Raise your feet.** Use your carry-on luggage as a footrest. Your back is under less strain when knees extend from your hips at a ninety-degree angle.

• **Tilt your seat back.** Lift your center of gravity with a comfortable lumbar support, taking pressure off your back and allowing the shoulders to relax naturally toward the floor. Review breathing and trunk positioning guidelines in Chapter Fourteen.

• **Provide adequate support for your head.** Try a neck pillow. These don't work for everyone, because of the unique curves in our backs, but they're relatively inexpensive and easy to find. Before you give up on a neck pillow, experiment with its turgidity. Reduce the air or remove a portion of the filling, to see if you can get it to feel just right.

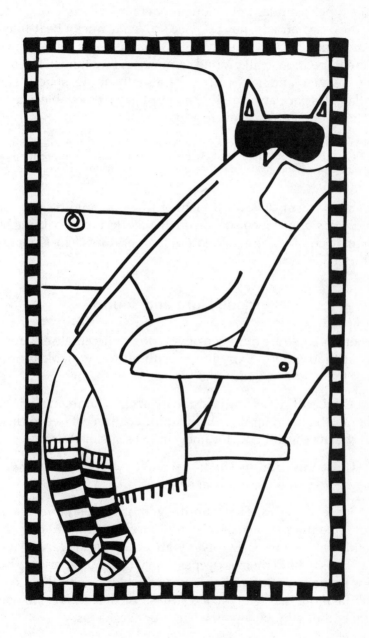

Shop thoughtfully: There is a wide variety of neck pillows on the market, including the more traditional U-shaped inflatable type, a similar but oblong model for leaning to one side or the other, and the newest fleece-covered, buckwheat-filled extravaganza called Bucky. Bucky claims to be miles above the competition in all-around comfort, and we think it is—but it's heavier and takes up substantially more space. The inflatables pack away easily, and most have removable, washable covers. Look for a warranty.

Bucky Travel and Leisure Pillows retail for about $25. Bucky Products, Inc., P.O. Box 31970, Seattle, WA 98103 (800/692-8259; fax: 206/545-0729). A variety of other neck pillows can be found in retail travel stores or through mail-order sources. See Appendix B.

▪ **Stay warm.** Ask for a blanket (there should be one for every passenger aboard). Slip on thick socks if you've brought them. See "Managing Volatile Temperatures" in Chapter Thirteen.

Blocking Light and Sound

Some people are more sensitive to their immediate environment than others. Experiment with all the variables. And don't scoff at eyeshades until you've tried them.

▪ **Click off your individual overhead lamp.** On night flights, the cabin lights will dim quite cozily. Feel free to click off the overhead lights for unoccupied seats in your row.

▪ **Close the window shade,** even if it's dark out. It may get light before you want to wake up.

▪ **Try eyeshades.** They run the gamut from simple, black poplin to fuschia, silk, and lacy. Be sure the ones you buy are comfortable to wear. Eyeshades are easily packable, and the darkness behind them is deeper than what you experience by closing your eyes. Eyeshades not only block light, they contribute more intangibly to a restful sense of solitude. No one will bother you when you wear your eyeshades.

▪ **Consider using earplugs or headphones.** See Chapter Fifteen for a full discussion.

Safeguarding Your Sanctity

If you want to sleep, it's important to let neighboring passengers and the flight attendants onboard know.

Wear those eyeshades. Eyeshades are a firm statement of intent and communicate the clear message that you don't want meals, magazines, or conversation. If you feel the need to be explicit, fashion a "Do Not Disturb" message with fabric tape and an indelible marker across the front.

On long trips, especially when you're crossing time zones and flying at night, fasten your seatbelt low around the hips *outside* your blanket or other top layer. This precaution will spare you being wakened by the flight attendant who, if there is turbulence or an intermediate stop, has to make sure your belt is fastened.

·17·

Prevent Motion Sickness

In the early days of commercial flight, traveling by air was horribly rough. The planes were smaller and much less mechanically sophisticated. Assaulted by movement and the noxious fumes that entered the cabin, over three-quarters of all passengers experienced full-blown nausea. Airlines carpeted their aircraft with rubber mats and furnished each traveler with a cardboard box for the inevitable vomiting.

Today's airplanes provide a smoother and more pleasant ride. There are still passengers, however, who are prone to experiencing motion sickness when they travel by air. Much more is known about the causes of motion sickness since those early days; queasy air travelers can now choose from a range of effective treatments, according to their individual symptoms and personal medicinal philosophy.

A Clash of the Senses

Current theory explains motion sickness as a clash of the senses. The eyes are busy telling the brain you are moving one way, while the vestibular system—the inner-ear apparatus that gives the brain information about movement and orientation—communicates a different message.

When the brain gets mixed messages, or when changes in information are too quick or extreme, you experience dizziness and nausea. Symptoms can also include headache, aversion to odors such as cigarette smoke or certain foods, cold sweats, heat rushes, sudden drowsiness, and pallor.

If you are the passenger in a car twisting along a serpentine mountain road, for example, the messages from your vestibular system may have trouble keeping up with the swift rate at which your eyes register changes in speed and direction. As a passenger, you have limited opportunity to anticipate change. It's markedly easier for the driver to prepare for dips and curves because he is in contact with, and in control of, the steering wheel.

Aboard an airplane, most visual clues indicate that you're sitting in a stationary room. The shifts in acceleration and direction registered by your vestibular system tell the brain a different story, and this conflict causes nausea.

There are no established guidelines that predict a tendency toward motion sickness. Researchers have noted that motion sickness increases with anxiety and heat exacerbates nausea. Motion sickness may also worsen with advanced age. Whoever you are, if you're going to be motion sick you'll probably have a little warning—dizziness, a headache, or mild queasiness, and extra saliva production before the active nausea.

It could be worse. Outside the earth's atmosphere, there is no alarm system. If an astronaut is prone toward motion sickness, she will vomit *instantaneously*, as soon as her eyes detect movement. Nor is there any reliable test she can take beforehand to predict the likelihood of experiencing motion sickness in space; our vestibular systems are built to navigate in a gravitational atmosphere.

On the earth, we know when motion sickness is coming and can take steps to prevent it. If you anticipate suffering from motion sickness, come prepared. There is a list of effective options. Which treatment is right for you? Only time and experimentation will tell. Combining the suggestions that follow with ginger helps most travelers, so we recommend starting there.

Staying Comfortable

For many passengers, lack of control during flight increases anxiety. Anxiety and fear exacerbate motion sickness, so the best thing you can do when you're feeling queasy is to get calm. Review the relaxation hints in Chapter Three. Keep an airsickness bag close by for reassurance. And do a few of these simple things to stay cool and comfortable:

- **Wear unrestrictive clothing.** Consider sweat suits, pajama-like clothing, or going without a bra or nylons.

- **Cool down.** Savor the ice of a cold drink. Splash your face with fresh, cool water. Aim the air nozzle directly on your face. Bathe in its blast.

- **Lean back. Close your eyes.** Because motion sickness is caused by a confusing overload of the senses, take steps to minimize the information coming in. You may experience a gentle drowsiness, one of the body's natural responses to nausea. Succumb.

- **Eat lightly** when you travel, *but do eat.* A totally empty stomach is just as bad as an overly full one. (Both an empty stomach and anxiety produce gas. The extra gas increases pressure on the stomach, heightening nausea. Small amounts of food provide an absorbent buffer.) As you snack, avoid gas-producing foods like apples and beans.

- **Avoid alcohol** during your flight and partake only moderately at dinner the night before. Alcohol usually makes motion sickness worse.

- **Avoid fizzy drinks.** Extra pressure from the gas of carbonation exacerbates nausea. Fruit juices, tea, or the bottled water you pack yourself are the most calming for your stomach. Of all tea options, hot peppermint tea is one of the best; peppermint is a gentle stomach soother, used after meals in many cultures. Take a few tea bags with you. The flight attendants will offer hot water but usually no herbal tea options. Peppermint in capsule form is also available for those who don't want to trouble with tea.

- **Sit in the middle of the plane,** over the wings, where the ride is the smoothest.

Medication Options

Make sure the treatment you choose is a good fit. If fear and anxiety are part of your flying experience, take them seriously. Work to reduce your anxiety, then tackle the motion sickness. This is not to say that motion sickness is an imaginary ailment; quite the contrary! We travel, we know. But heading straight for the pharmacy may blur contributing issues. You can start addressing your discomfort by turning back to the program in Chapter Three. The information on medication options will be here, waiting and ready when you are.

Ginger

Yes, ginger. You may already use this zappy spice for cooking. Ginger powder, made by drying and pulverizing the plant's unpeeled root, has been instrumental in Chinese medicine for thousands of years. Dried ginger has been used to treat conditions ranging from stomach ailments and nausea to inflammation of the joints. It's not known for sure how it works, but some researchers believe that it interferes with the brain's release of the stress hormones epinephrine and norepinephrine to the stomach, which causes queasiness.

Because it is an anti-inflammatory and promotes elimination of intestinal gas and soothes the gastrointestinal tract, ginger reduces symptoms associated with motion sickness, including dizziness, nausea, vomiting, and cold sweating. The average dose is 1,000 to 1,500 milligrams, a half hour to an hour before scheduled takeoff. Continue as needed.

Powdered ginger for making your own capsules can be found in any cooking spice section. Empty gelatin capsules can be purchased in health food stores. Prepacked capsules are available in the food supplement section of most health food stores. Unabashed gnawing of the root is also an option—but you'll have to chew a lot of it. There are other useful ginger options: chocolate-covered candied ginger, chewy ginger candies, and hard ginger lozenges. Look for the latter two in an Asian grocery store.

Dramamine

Many people who suffer from motion sickness depend on Dramamine. And this over-the-counter medication makes most of them feel extremely drowsy. Dramamine is available in both pill and chewable tablet form. Beware: Anything that makes you drowsy will interfere with your ability to adapt to the stress of travel, changing time zones, and new environmental conditions. Armies of former Dramamine users are being "liberated" by the equally if not more effective use of ginger capsules.

Wristbands

Used most notably by the British navy in the 1800s, wristbands work to prevent motion sickness by applying a small but steady amount of pressure to the *nei-kuan* acupressure point on the inside of the wrist. Two popular brand names are Sea Band and MorningGarde. They look like slender cotton sweatbands, and have one slightly cone-shaped plastic knob on the inner side. Wear a band on each wrist with the knob placed between your flexor tendons, a distance of three fingers' width above the crease of your wrist. They work best if you press the button every so often. Most are relatively inexpensive and washable. Wristbands last until you lose them or the elastic wears out.

Ear Patches

Ear patches are extremely popular among deep-sea fishers. Available by prescription only, an ear patch is a medicated adhesive circle (about the size of a dime) from which your skin slowly absorbs one of several active ingredients that block signals from the inner ear and quiet the stomach. Users place a patch behind one of their ears for protection from nausea for up to seventy-two hours.

According to a number of patients and physicians, the ear patches using the active ingredient scopolamine are the most effective and cause the least drowsiness. Other possible side effects include blurred vision, dryness of the mouth, and disorientation. Use this medication only under the guidance of a doctor and, as with all therapies, do try a patch before your trip so side effects are no surprise.

Beta Blockers

These medications are not prescribed for motion sickness per se but for the extreme anxiety that can cause motion sickness. Common for the treatment of high blood pressure and heart problems, beta blockers are also used by many professional performers to combat stage fright. They work by decreasing the "fight or flight" response. One of the original beta blockers is Inderal (the generic name is propranolol). Available by prescription only, beta blockers may cause drowsiness, mild dizziness, or lightheadedness.

Airbag Etiquette

There is an unnecessary sense of shame associated with using an airsickness bag. Passengers feel mortified when they vomit, even when they do so into the convenient, low-profile receptacle provided exactly for that purpose.

Feeling nauseated is no fun, and vomiting can be messy. But don't increase your own anxiety by worrying about what other people will think. Use your bag, and don't be embarrassed to ask for your seatmate's if you need it. Feel free to summon a flight attendant and request a damp cloth or glass of ice. When you're able, go to the lavatory; bathe your face, neck, and hands in cool water. These simple acts will help you regain your bearings and your pride.

What to do with the used bag? Fold or roll the top of your bag down onto itself, and throw it away in the bathroom depository marked For Trash. If you feel more comfortable staying seated, or don't feel comfortable walking with a used bag, close it up tightly and tuck it into the seatback pocket in front of you. Ask a flight attendant as you leave if he could help you by disposing of the bag. A little courage, honesty, and dignified appreciation are what's appropriate here.

·18·

How to Deal with Difficult Passengers

D ifficult passengers are those who—for whatever reason and no matter how—are behaving in a way that keeps you from getting what you need during your flight. There are several different schools of thought concerning how best to deal with them.

Employing Social Cues

The first is what we'll call the "school of indirect communication." The most amusing suggestion along this line—and probably the most effective—comes from a nun who spends a good deal of her time on long international flights. When she feels like a nearby passenger is becoming invasive, physically or conversationally, she employs this forbidding strategy: She reaches for her airsickness bag and holds it to her mouth. If imminent vomit isn't enough to warn him off, she will turn to her bothersome seatmate and say, "I don't think one bag is going to be enough. May I have yours?"

Avoid eye contact, turn your body away from the offending individual, answer questions in monosyllables, become engrossed in a magazine. Simply closing one's eyes, travelers agree, is not always enough to communicate a boundary. To establish personal space, you need to set clear limits from the outset: Create an aura that says you have something else to do. Be less friendly, make minimal small talk. Be polite without engaging.

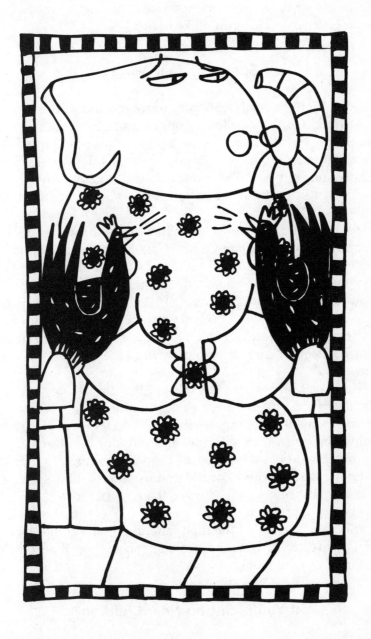

Eyeshades send definite don't-bother-me signals, as do headphones and earplugs. Combine eyeshades with a pair of earplugs, and you're impenetrable. The flight attendants won't even ask what you'd like to drink.

Speaking Your Mind

Your highly social seatmate, however, may lie in wait, watching breathlessly for an opportunity to break in once you've had a little nap. This brings us to "the academy of direct communication," an approach that is definitely more challenging but, we believe, ultimately the most satisfying. By being truthful about what you need, you stand the best chance of getting it.

Your communication doesn't have to be brutal, rude, or snappy. Be respectful and frank. Use "I" statements: "I hope you have a good flight. I'd rather not talk while we're in the air, but am going to [read my book, meditate on this month's horoscope, work on a project, etc.]." Any violation can calmly and firmly be met with: "When you [ask questions, point out exciting land features, etc.], I have a hard time concentrating. I'm glad you're enjoying the view, but I really don't want to talk."

The situation usually doesn't get this far. When you articulate the desire to be left alone without being apologetic, without creating the impression that you'll be available for conversation in a little while, and without belittling your seatmate, you get the peace and sanctity you're after right from the start. If your seatmate understands that the solitude you want has more to do with you than any flaw of his, he will probably participate in making sure you get it. "Shhh...," you'll hear him say to the flight attendant who comes by as you try to doze. "I think she just wants some quiet time. Don't disturb her with that snack pack, okay?"

If You're Sitting Near Children

When a restless child invades your space, kicking the back of your seat or repeatedly snapping the ashtray open and closed, speak to him about it. Treat him like an equal, explaining how what he's doing affects you and how you feel about that. Children respond best when you give them an alternative: "How about asking the flight attendant if she has any crayons or cards?" If you feel hesitant to do this, or do it and get no constructive response, go ahead and ask the child's parents—or the flight attendant when children are traveling alone—to address the child's behavior.

A crying child is the best argument for earplugs. Even if you've never used them and don't think you will, we encourage you to take a pair on your next trip. The plugs don't take up much room, nor are they heavy. They just might make the difference between protracted misery and rest. If the situation becomes desperate, request a seat change.

If what you're looking for is a quiet, peaceful trip, don't start a conversation with a child traveling alone. Young people tend to have a more difficult time understanding shifting boundaries—when you're available, when you're not— especially if they have to be persistent to get attention at home. Unless you're willing to take the child under your wing, it's best to let her attach herself to a flight attendant right from the start. It'll be easier on all of you.

Fly Defensively

The world is full of dangerous things. There are tiny pathogens and men with guns. There is eating and bathing and driving through the neighborhood. If we thought about all the things that could happen to us in a given day, we'd never get out of bed.

We cope with this panorama of risks and threats by shutting out some and selectively focusing on others. You may be reading this book because you're one of the many who selectively focus on flying—even though it is the safest mode of vehicular transportation. If so, you may be prone to ignoring safety precautions and tuning out safety information for fear that paying attention to safety will only increase your apprehension.

Don't. *Paying attention to safety doesn't have to create a sense of alarm.* Treat flying like you would anything else.

If you took a glass-bottom-boat cruise into the Okefenokee Swamp, you would wear a life jacket. Crossing the street, you look both ways before stepping off the curb. You probably keep emergency numbers by the phone at home. Flying calls for no more than the same precautionary common sense you would use to protect your safety in other situations .

The numbers indicate that frequent flyers are better able to take care of themselves in emergencies; researchers assume this is because regular travelers are more familiar with aircraft than other passengers, and they panic less. You can achieve both the familiarity and the calm, no matter how many times you've been in the air.

▪ **Listen to the flight emergency procedures review** at the beginning of the flight. Make sure you understand the tasks outlined, including the opening and closing of your safety belt, breathing through the auxiliary oxygen mask, and pulling out your seat cushion for floating. If anything seems confusing, consult the laminated safety procedure card in the seatback pocket in front of you. Summon a flight attendant after takeoff if you have additional questions.

▪ **Look over at the emergency exit closest to you.** Count the number of seat rows between you and it, figure out how you'd get to the door if cabin lights were dim or out. Take a minute to study the diagrams on the safety card that show how to open the door, noting that the door first opens *inward*. Imagine opening it in the dark.

▪ **Be familiar with the brace position.** Consult the diagram on the safety card for a clear example.

▪ **Don't panic** if you experience something unusual. Don't stand up or barrage the flight attendant with questions; let everyone on the crew do their job. If and when passengers are given instructions, follow them calmly.

▪ **Keep your safety belt fastened** low and tight around your hips during takeoff, landing, and whenever you are seated— even when the sign has been turned off.

Is it possible to choose a safe flight? Well, yes. No matter what flight you choose, your chances of arriving unharmed are superb. You may, however, want to avoid flying in countries where regulation is less stringent. A comparison of airline safety records around the world shows significant differences: air travel in wealthier countries tends to be safer than air travel in poorer countries. Book major international carriers whenever possible. If in doubt, ask your travel agent to research the safety records of the airlines you plan to use. Keep in mind that there is no country in the world in which, statistically, it's safer to drive than to fly.

TIP Call the State Department's traveler's advisory center (202/647-5225) or its automated fax service (202/647-3000) for a current report on transportation safety for the country or countries in which you intend to fly. If general country warnings are appropriate, you'll find them there.

Another area that bears special consideration is flying on small commuter airplanes. While the flight safety records of major U.S. carriers are all excellent, the larger, regularly scheduled commercial aircraft have a slightly better safety record than small commuter airplanes.

If you want to speak to a live human being about U.S. airplane safety standards, call the FAA's toll-free Consumer Safety Hotline (800/255-1111) and ask for the number of a Flight Standards District Office in your area. Personnel at the Standards District Offices are responsible for monitoring airlines' adherence to their FAA-mandated safety and maintenance programs. They are usually more than willing to discuss aircraft safety with callers. If you experience airplane conditions or airline personnel behavior that you feel is unsafe, make a report to the Consumer Safety Hotline at the same toll-free number. The FAA investigators will pursue your concern within thirty days.

·20·

Know Your Rights

Since the deregulation of the airline industry under President Reagan, your options in the case of delays and cancellations on U.S. carriers vary from airline to airline based on the contract you enter into by purchasing your ticket. Only in the case of overbooking do you have rights guaranteed by law.

Contract? Yes, it is a contract, sometimes referred to as "conditions of carriage." In the U.S., the Department of Transportation (DOT) requires that your ticket contain or refer to this contract. U.S. carriers must keep complete copies at their ticket offices and airport counters; you can also request free copies by mail. International airlines operate under different regulations but are usually required to keep a copy of what are called "tariff rules" at city and airport ticket offices.

The DOT rules also dictate that your ticket—or the materials with it—state all terms that restrict refunds, impose financial penalties, or allow the airline to raise the ticket price after purchase. If an airline agent insists that your ticket is nonrefundable, for example, but neither the ticket nor materials with it say so, then it is fully refundable.

TIP If the airline fails to abide by its contractual or statutory obligations, make a complaint to the DOT. Send a letter and copies of all applicable correspondence to: Consumer Affairs Division, Room 10405, Office of Community and Consumer Affairs, Department of Transportation, 400 7th Street S.W., Washington, DC 20590 (202/366-2220). Be sure to note your daytime telephone number.

In the interest of providing good customer service, most airlines extend themselves beyond what is required by law or contract. Every airline has its own policies for dealing with delays, mix-ups, and passenger predicaments. Unfortunately, these are not always made clear to passengers. Experience and perseverance are the only ways to discover the full breadth of the benefits available to you.

Adopt the attitude that everything is open to negotiation. If the ticket agent behind the counter doesn't have the authority to grant the request you believe is fair, keep asking until you find the person who does. Be reasonable and be appreciative. Charm and diplomacy will take you much further than threats or ill-tempered demands.

Bring to bear everything you know about human psychology. Step into the airline official's shoes. What would make you want to be helpful?

Avoid placing blame while asking for help (at least initially). Tell the ticket agent how you're feeling: "I'm very worried." Explain your situation clearly: "I'm going to miss my connecting flight, and I can't afford a hotel if I have to stay overnight." Then ask: "I'm wondering if there's any way you could...." Be specific. Ask for what you want, knowing that you may have to settle for less.

We recommend the booklet *Facts & Advice for Airline Passengers.* Including subjects such as "How to Find the Best Air Fare," "Airline Bankruptcies and You," and "Constructive Complaining," it can be purchased for $5 from: Aviation Consumer Action Project, P.O. Box 19029, Washington, DC 20036 (202/638-4000).

Delays

If your flight is delayed, ask an airline representative about the cause. If the delay is the fault of the airline (mechanical complications, for example) and total delay time is an hour or more, most airlines will bend over backwards to get you on the next available flight, with no extra fare or change fee— even if it means putting you in first class. Be sure the airline causing the delay will absorb any additional costs *before* you accept these new arrangements.

Some are only willing to reroute you on *their* next available flight. When the delay is beyond the airline's control (weather, war, earthquake, etc.), they're less likely to help out beyond contractual requirements. If your life savings or your reputation hinge on making a meeting, fly in the day before.

Most airlines will provide a full refund (even if your ticket is marked nonrefundable) if they are not able to arrange a reasonable substitute flight. Under some contracts, you can claim a full refund if the substitute is not acceptable to you.

TIP Anyone who flies frequently or has the time would be well advised to write for conditions of carriage for the airlines with which they travel. Zero in on what the airline offers in the event of a "schedule irregularity."

If you're afraid a delay will cause you to miss a connecting flight, get prepared:

▪ While you're still on the airplane, use the airline magazine or an OAG *Pocket Flight Guide* to **review the layout of the airport.** How far away is the gate for your next flight? Avoid security lines wherever possible. Plot a course of action and get ready to sprint.

▪ **Notify airline personnel as soon as you can.** They may provide a custom shuttle to the connecting gate or, especially if there are other passengers similarly affected, ask the connecting flight to wait.

TIP Don't rely on a monitor's report that your flight has already left. Flight status is usually listed according to *scheduled*, not *actual*, departure times. If you're within minutes, run ahead to the gate. The flight may still be boarding.

Cancellations

Canceled flights are handled in the same manner as delays. Most airlines will do their utmost to rebook you on the next plane scheduled; if they can't arrange a reasonable alternative, the full purchase price of your ticket will be refunded.

TIP Your travel agent may suggest you combine two separate round-trip tickets to secure a better fare. You should be aware that if delay or cancellation of the first flight makes you miss the second, the earlier carrier has no responsibility to reroute you—even if both tickets are with the same airline—although they may be kind enough to do so. Your entire trip must be written *on one ticket* to gain maximum assistance from the airline at fault.

As soon as you know a flight is canceled, take steps to re-book. Don't wait in line; head directly for a telephone booth. Call the airline's toll-free reservations number and make a reservation on the next available flight. *Then* go stand in line to have your old ticket endorsed for use on the new flight.

TIP If a delay, cancellation, or other airline snafu means you have to stay overnight at your own expense, ask an airline official to call nearby hotels and secure a "distressed passenger rate" for you. If they can't or won't, explain the circumstances to the hotel manager in person. Some travel insurance policies, purchased separately or furnished as a benefit of charging tickets on some credit cards, provide reimbursement for expenses incurred as a result of delay.

Overbooking

With increasing frequency, airlines are overbooking their flights. Usually, a significant number of the passengers with reservations don't show. If too many passengers check in, the first thing the gate agent will do is ask for volunteers. Before "bumping" anyone involuntarily, DOT rules require that U.S. commercial carriers first seek willing passengers. If the call goes out and you're traveling on a flexible schedule, you may want to stand up and be compensated.

Voluntary Bumping

There is no limit to the amount of compensation volunteers can receive. The greater the pressure, the larger the prize. Agents are obliged to start negotiating with the bare minimum: perhaps a $150 flight certificate and standby status on a later flight. Many a gate audience has been amused to watch offerings rise, much to the chagrin of initial volunteers. To wait is to gamble.

If you decide to relinquish your seat, make sure you know exactly what you'll get in return.

▪ **Decide how flexible you can be before you give up your ticket.** When is the next available flight? Would you have a guaranteed reservation, or have to fly standby? What would your status be on subsequent connecting flights?

- **Make sure you don't end up spending as much as, or even more than, you gain.** Will the airline provide free meals while you wait for the next flight? Phone calls? Transport? A hotel room if needed?

- **Read the extra-fine print** on the proffered flight certificate before accepting it. Are there any travel restrictions, blackout dates? Consider whether or not you can take more vacation time before the expiration date. Does the voucher guarantee a reservation, or a standby slot?

Involuntary Bumping

If the airline has overbooked your flight and there aren't enough volunteers, watch out. The last passengers to the gate are usually the first to be bumped, even if they already have seat assignments and boarding passes. When your travel plans are urgent, the best defense is to allow plenty of time for gate check-in.

Most airline conditions of carriage provide the same re-routing benefits as they do for delays and cancellations. In addition, DOT regulations guarantee you the following as a minimum:

- **A written statement** explaining your rights and how the airline decides who gets seats in the case of overbooking.

- **Nothing else,** if the airline manages to get you on a flight and to your destination within one hour of previously scheduled arrival time (on one of their planes or anyone else's).

- **The value of a one-way fare to your final destination—** up to $200—if substitute transportation is arranged to deliver you between one and two hours of your original flight. The airline may offer a free flight coupon for the same amount, but *whether you take the money or the voucher is up to you.*

- **Two hundred percent of the one-way fare to your final destination**—up to $400—if substitute transportation is arranged to deliver you more than two hours after your original flight would have (four hours for international flights). Again, the airline may offer a free flight coupon for the same amount. *It is your right to choose.*

Some airlines' conditions of carriage provide benefits more generous than the DOT minimum. Investigate before you settle.

You are entitled to your check and/or free flight voucher on the spot (or within twenty-four hours if on the spot isn't convenient for *you*). Airline personnel may also have the authority to provide complimentary meals, hotel rooms, phone calls, etc., to insistent passengers. Be assertive about what you believe is fair.

If you accept compensation as offered, the deal is done. If, however, you feel the payment doesn't cover the loss you suffer as a result of being bumped, you can turn it down and negotiate with the airline's complaint department for more money; remember, the amounts described above are the DOT's *minimum* requirements. You can even file suit in state court against the airline, but be forewarned: Inconvenience and lost time aren't likely to be reimbursed.

The DOT rules only cover those passengers holding confirmed reservations on a domestic or outbound international, regularly scheduled, commercial flight (on a plane seating sixty passengers or more), with a U.S. carrier. If you're on a U.S. carrier between two foreign cities or entering the U.S., however, don't be afraid to ask! The airline may extend domestic policies in the name of good customer service.

To qualify for compensation under the DOT's rules, you must meet the airline's deadline for ticket purchase and fulfill the airline's requirements for check-in. Ask for an explanation of airline check-in requirements whenever you buy a ticket. Compensation is not required if you are bumped because a smaller plane was substituted for safety or operations reasons.

On non-U.S. airlines you may get more, or less, than with U.S. carriers. Look to individual carrier contracts and the laws of that airline's country of origin to know what to expect.

·21·

Make the Most of Your Layovers

Flyers groan when they scan down their itineraries and see three hours in Dallas, two in Philadelphia, or seven in Los Angeles. In most cases, travel agents can be resourceful and schedule tighter connections so that the layover, if any, is minimized. But when the connection's just not there or if a flight is delayed, you may find yourself sitting in the airport with extra time on your hands. *Enjoy it.* That layover may turn out to be a very pleasing part of your flight.

Stashing the Heavies

Before doing anything else, you'll want to free yourself of any cumbersome carry-ons. If you are a first- or business-class passenger or a member of an airline lounge, you can leave your bags there. Be warned, however, that you do this at your own risk; there is generally no attendant on watch.

Anyone can use a few quarters and rent a locker; just ask at the information booth or a ticket counter to find out if there are lockers in the airport, and where.

If you're planning on staying in one general area, you can use a light, retractable cable lock to secure your luggage to a nearby chair leg. If the cable lock isn't slender enough to run through main zipper holes, we recommend using a small combination or key lock to do so and then running the cable through it. Any valuables should be kept with you, or at least packed deep inside the bag.

We recommend Eagle Creek's retractable cable lock. It looses a forty-two-inch (120 cm) steel cable from a compact and resetable three-dial lock; retail price is around $15. See Appendix B for ordering information.

When leaving luggage isn't an option, at least rent a luggage cart. Usually costing under $2 and available in most larger airports, a cart will lighten the load and give your arms a break. If the main building is fresh out of wheels, scope the baggage carousels and loading curbs.

Sleuthing Airport Conveniences

Airports are fascinating places to be. The only prerequisite for adventure is a good attitude. Besides offering prime people-watching, airports often sponsor art shows and special exhibits. If you have enough time to leave the airport, there are even more possibilities.

In addition to the usual realm of shops with their sweatshirts and magazines, you may find a few surprises. The new Denver airport boasts a seven-and-a-half million dollar art collection. Bahrain International Airport is one of a growing number that offers travelers the service of a twenty-four-hour bank. The airport in Portland, Oregon, hosts a range of intriguing specialty shops, all required to charge prices equal to those at nonairport locations.

Several airports offer back and face massages. Look for a health club. Many airports have shower facilities available for a nominal fee. Larger airports, and even some of the smaller ones, have hair salons and postal services. You could have your shoes shined, get a spontaneous pedicure, or send postcards to all those relatives you've been meaning to write.

Don't worry about exchanging currency in a foreign airport; major credit cards are almost always accepted for payment. If you feel drawn to shop in a duty-free store, be aware that the prices inside are not necessarily bargains; tax savings are often offset by inflated airport prices.

If you want to use the time to make phone calls, take a list of phone numbers (or messages to return) in your carry-on. In addition to carrying a pocketful of coins or calling collect, there are now more convenient—and cheaper—methods.

Credit cards: One convenient way to call long distance (or local) is to use a phone that takes a credit card. Most airports have them. You'll be billed with the next credit card statement. *Calling cards:* You can avoid operator charges by using a telephone company calling card—either at a phone designated specifically for that purpose, or by punching in the required numbers at any phone.

Using your calling card outside the U.S. is sometimes more complicated. Your best bet is to access your company's English-speaking operator directly using a designated phone or a specific access number. Most major phone companies provide billfold-size guides with step-by-step instructions. Otherwise, you'll have to go through a local operator—more expensive and less handy.

If you're looking for a quiet place to read, work, or think, ask if there is an airport chapel. Chapels are more common than you might expect, and infinitely more peaceful than the main buildings.

If you want to use the extra time to sleep, ask around to find out if any of the observation or seating areas are conducive to stretching out. Don't assume every seat in the airport is narrow with permanent armrests. Some airports even have mini-hotels in them, offering beds by the half-hour for a reasonable price.

Until recently, airport food has been fairly dismal. There seems to be a trend, however, toward more variety, better quality, and healthier offerings. Don't assume that what you see is all there is. Find out if there's a fruit stand, a "food court," or a fine restaurant somewhat removed from the terminal's hustle-bustle. Don't settle for the hot dog until you're well apprised of all the options.

Airport clubs are an option you may want to explore. Geared primarily toward the business traveler, airport clubs tend to be posh and austere. They're also very comfortable and stocked with conveniences. Services vary from airline to airline, and from location to location. There's usually a bar and tall windows for looking out over the runway, television, fax machines, modem ports, desks, outlets for laptop computers, and phones on which local calls are free. In an airport club, you'll be served free soda, snacks, and sometimes espresso. Tables are casually stacked with current newspapers and magazines. Airport club personnel support business travelers with other services, including handling flight reservations and ticketing, check-in (for passengers without luggage), car rental, and other same-day travel details. More than anything else, airport clubs are blissfully, restfully quiet.

Airlines grant club access to their passengers who are flying first or business class, or to any passenger for an annual fee; ask an airline representative about membership. The fee charged by most airlines is not prohibitive. Delta, for example, sells memberships to its Crown Club lounges for $150 a year. Membership to United's Red Carpet Rooms cost $275, including the initiation fee.

If you have several hours at your disposal, you may want to leave the airport. A visitor's bureau or tourist's wall stocked with brochures is a good way to learn a bit about the area. Don't be bashful about asking airport personnel for recommendations.

How about a hotel near the airport? It may have an outdoor pool, an indoor pool, a gym, sauna, or whirlpool. Day-use passes are often available for these amenities, and the shuttle back and forth is free (but tipping is appropriate).

The "fastest, cheapest, and most convenient" routes to and from almost four hundred airport terminals around the world are laid out in *Salk's International Airport Transit Guide* ($7.95). See Appendix B for retail and mail-order sources. Among more extravagant options—like chartering a helicopter—are useful, practical shortcuts.

There is often a shuttle that runs, free of charge, to the closest downtown area. If not, take a public bus—inexpensive and colorful. Hotel vans will also run you to the city for the price of a good tip. You can explore a new city, visit a museum, or just ride around and come back. Make sure you can get back to the airport and safely to the gate on time for your flight. Check the schedule carefully *before* you leave. A mistake could mean an outrageous taxi fare or the change fee and inconvenience of booking another flight.

To find out what your options are ahead of time, call the airport and ask for information or public affairs. The folks at the other end can describe their facilities and anything of interest around the airport. Your travel agent can look up local highlights to make a few sight-seeing suggestions. Most

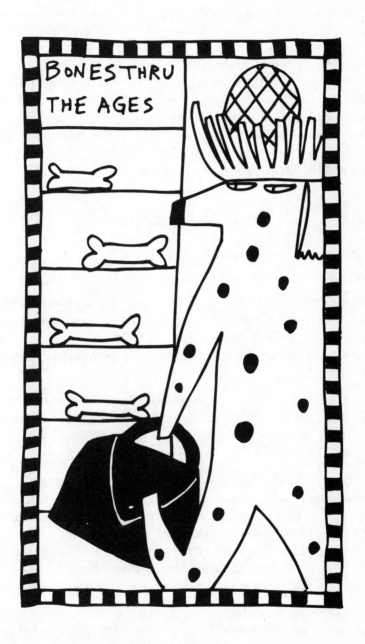

travel agents have an up-to-date copy of the Official Airline Guides (OAG) *Travel Planner* in the office, which contains maps of airport layouts and listings of nearby attractions. You can buy your own *Travel Planner* if you like, but the yearly subscription rate is about $130 and many of the pages are devoted to car rental advertising.

In the air, leaf through an airline magazine. Sandwiched between the shopping section and ads, these publications feature airport layouts, tourist information and other inviting particulars. Once you're in the airport, ask at the information desk, look at a terminal map, or just head down a concourse toward the main terminal to find out what's there.

Conducting Business

Take what you need to do good work during and between flights.

▪ Pack your planner or calendar/organizer so it's accessible, and use your time to outline projects, assign the steps, make useful lists. Do paperwork. Fill out expense forms. Take industry reading or the stack of articles you keep meaning to review.

▪ Take "ditchables": Make photocopies of documents you need to review, leaving the originals in your office. You can dump them when you're through, lightening your load from layover to layover.

▪ Mail or FedEx papers back to yourself. Take company air bills along in your briefcase and send finished work from the airport. Call ahead to the airport where you have a scheduled layover to ask which express mail carrier services are in the terminal and where that carrier's drop box is located. If you use regular mail, take enough of your own stamps to send the package. Wall-mounted dispensers are often empty.

▪ Use layover or delay time to call the office, check your voicemail, or keep the ball rolling on projects. Although there are phones on most airplanes, it's best to use them only for delivering messages. Don't count on a connection clear enough for a two-way conversation. Let the other party know that they can hear you better than you can hear them: "I can't hear you very well, so I'm just going to have to talk. If you need to respond, please leave me a voicemail and I'll check my messages during the Reno layover, at 4 o'clock E.S.T."

▪ Find out if there is an "office center" you can access; many airports offer them. Facilities include fax machines, modems, copiers, printers, and conference rooms, all for use at fairly reasonable fees. Some airports contain little offices for rent by the hour that can be used for meetings or for private work. They are usually equipped with both phone and fax.

▪ Be realistic. Inventory the list of tasks you have to do, ask yourself what materials you can reasonably work with, and check everything else with your luggage. If you haul too much around with you, the extra weight and defeating immensity of work left unfinished will prove more frustrating than productive.

Who knows? You may plan layovers so efficiently that the solitary time in the air can be used simply to *think*. Rolling an issue around in your mind, without a definite agenda, often leads to unusually creative solutions.

·22·

Avoid Jet Lag

President Lyndon Johnson coped with jet lag by forcing the rest of the world to adopt his own clock. No matter where around the globe he traveled, he scheduled meetings on White House time—even if it meant dinner at 2 A.M. While this may have worked for the president, it probably isn't very practical for the rest of us.

The term *jet lag* describes a bundle of uncomfortable physical symptoms—extreme fatigue and sleep disturbance, loss of con-centration, general disorientation, impaired judgment, gastrointestinal upset—that result when your body clock is out of synch with the clock on the wall. Jet lag gets worse with age and is a particular problem for travelers who are sleep deprived already.

Your Body's Internal Clock

The human clock progresses in a series of roughly twenty-four-hour cycles. These cycles are called "circadian," from the Latin *circa*, about, and *dien*, meaning day. Our circadian rhythms coordinate most noticeably with the daily intervals of light and darkness. This happens not only in humans (and mammals); the daily four-hour opening of a morning glory is also timed by a circadian clock.

Would humans maintain their twenty-four-hour cycles without the cues of night and day? Probably. Research indicates that approximately one-half of all sight-impaired and many fully sighted individuals, not responding biochemically to the difference between light and dark, settle naturally into a twenty-five-hour clock. A series of experiments spurred by the 1969 adventure of Jacques Chabert, a twenty-three-year-old Frenchman who spent half a year at 60° Centigrade and 100 percent humidity in a cave sixty-five meters below the earth's surface, also indicates that humans have a twenty-four- to twenty-five-hour sleep cycle.

We know, then, that sunlight doesn't determine the length of the cycle. Natural outdoor light, however, even if muted by clouds, does communicate with the body about *when to start* each cycle. This may be why many people have a harder time getting out of bed in the winter when sunrise comes later, and why some people feel drowsy if they stay inside on dark days. (Ordinary indoor lighting has no effect on your internal clock.)

Your body will naturally adjust to time changes at a rate of one hour per day. How can you adapt more quickly to local time?

Tips for Easier Adjustment

Adjustment is easier for travelers flying east to west, because it's less stressful for the body to incorporate an initially longer day. When you fly from Seattle to Paris, however, night comes earlier. That ritual morning croissant is going to come quite a bit earlier than you expect; about eight hours earlier, in fact, or a little more than an average night's sleep. To encourage the successful reorientation of your body clock, you'll want to:

• Approach air travel in as **rested and healthy** a state as you possibly can.

• **Avoid alcohol** and other depressants (such as motion sickness medications and other drugs that cause drowsiness).

• **Keep your body comfortable** using the techniques and travel aids that work best for you.

• **Eat lighter** than normal before and during flight. Charles Lindberg was well advised; he ate only one sandwich during the thirty-four hours of his famous 1927 transatlantic solo flight. After landing, feel free to fill up on local fare.

▪ **Adopt destination time** as soon as you step on the plane. Do everything you can to encourage your body to stick to it. Don't ask yourself, "What time is it, *really*?"

▪ **Don't sleep in.** If a nap is absolutely crucial to survival, limit yourself to an hour.

▪ **Stay warm.** Because body temperature fluctuates like clockwork (pun intended), you'll find, in new time zones, that you're cold at odd times of the day. Be prepared, keeping yourself comfortable and healthy.

Consult your doctor about adjusting your schedule for time-sensitive medication you may be taking, like estrogen, birth control pills, heart medication or antidepressants.

TIP Crafty business travelers use jet lag to their advantage by scheduling meetings when they're freshest—and others are lagging. Journeying west to east, negotiate complicated deals over a late dinner meeting. Theoretically, this strategy would be most effective in the day or two following arrival, while you're still on home time and *before* other jet lag symptoms set in.

Method I : Signaling with Melatonin

The pineal gland, once called the "seat of the soul" by sixteenth-century philosopher René Descartes, was long considered by the Western medical community to be a useless organ. More recently, however, scientists have discovered that this gland, found nestled in the forebrain, is responsible for the body's daily production of the hormone melatonin.

Among other things, melatonin induces sleep. The production of melatonin is suppressed by daylight; as darkness falls, melatonin is released from the pineal gland into the body's blood stream and cues the sleep cycle to begin. Studies show that melatonin not only begins this cycle but improves overall sleep quality.

In addition to being used for the treatment of insomnia, melatonin has proved to be a tremendously effective aid in reducing jet lag. It may actually cut adjustment to new time zones by half. No researcher in the field, one scientist laughed, would dream of traveling to an international conference without it. Melatonin, taken about two hours before bed, clues your body in to the fact that night is happening earlier.

To use melatonin successfully: When you land, get outside for a walk if at all possible. At least do some stretches and good breathing, stay active, and stay awake. You're on local time now. Two hours before you normally go to sleep (again, using *local* clocks), take the appropriate dose of melatonin. Set your alarm to wake you the next morning, and continue. Get outside in the sunlight during the day, stay active, then take your melatonin two hours before bedtime. Note that there is no added benefit gained from beginning melatonin before arrival time; such use may, in fact, cause extra drowsiness.

The number of time zones you've crossed, divided by two, will give you a rough idea how many days to use the capsules. But pay attention to your body. If you wake up drowsy, stop. You have arrived.

Synthetic melatonin is nonaddictive and nontoxic. If you have questions or concerns, ask your doctor or pharmacist. You can get it at your local health food store, from a nutritional pharmaceutical, through your physician or from a mail-order distributor. The average dose is three to nine milligrams before bedtime. Pharmacists recommend trying this before you travel to see how your body reacts to it. If you take too much, you'll feel drowsy the day after.

Ecological Formulas retails a bottle of 60 three-milligram capsules for $16.95, plus $1.50 shipping: 1061 B. Shary Circle, Concord, CA 94518 (800/888-4585 or 510/827-2636).

Method II : The Anti–Jet Lag Diet

A different approach to the problem comes from the U.S. Department of Energy's Argonne National Laboratory. Scientists there, led by Dr. Charles F. Ehret, have compiled their own list of influences on the human body clock: light and dark, social cues such as meal times, natural chemicals like caffeine, and *timing*. (Body chemistry changes substantially over its twenty-four-hour course; "timing" refers to the impact of different factors on the body during different stages of the day.)

Two of the primary keys to combating jet lag, Argonne scientists maintain, lie in the body's storage organs for energy reserves (including the muscles and the liver), and the production of glycogen (which is, essentially, the fuel of the human body). When glycogen reserves are allowed to run low through absolute fasting or light eating, we become extra sensitive to the effects of light and darkness, food, and methylated xanthines. Caffeine is one of these; theobromine, found in chocolate, is another.

The Argonne scientists suggest using these factors in combinations that seem to boot the body clock forward to a new time frame. Although the schedule in its entirety may seem complicated, it does produce results for many.

Some travelers find it too difficult to follow this regime to the letter, but do find that incorporating even some elements aids adjustment. For example, many swear by light eating before and during flight, then loading up on carbohydrates upon arrival for a good night's sleep. We offer a streamlined version of the Argonne Anti–Jet Lag Diet here.

Preflight

Determine the customary breakfast time at your final destination. Count back: your day of arrival, plus one travel day, plus three full days at home before takeoff. This is the day to begin.

Starting on this day, eat meals according to your normal schedule. On day one, FEAST: eat heartily with high-protein breakfast and lunch, then a high-carbohydrate dinner. Don't drink coffee (or other caffeinated beverages like tea and cola) except in the late afternoon, between 3 and 5 P.M.

On day two, FAST with a day of light meals: salads, light soups, fruits, and juices. Again, no coffee—except between 3 and 5 P.M.

On day three, FEAST again.

Inflight

On day four, departure day, FAST. If you are including caffeinated beverages in your regimen, drink them in the morning if traveling west, or between 6 and 11 P.M. if traveling east. While flying, avoid alcohol. If the flight is long enough, sleep until normal breakfast time at your destination, *but no later.*

Postflight

FEAST upon landing. Stay awake, and stay active. Do as the locals do; continue the day's meals, if there are any left, according to the regular meal times in your destination time zone.

Making Sense of the Regimen

High-protein feasts stimulate the body's active cycle. Suitable high-protein feasts include steak, eggs, hamburgers, high-protein cereals, and green beans.

High-carbohydrate feasts stimulate sleep. These include spaghetti and other pastas (but not meatballs!), crepes (again, no meat filling), potatoes and other starchy vegetables, and sweet desserts.

Fast days help deplete the liver's store of carbohydrates, thereby preparing the body's clock for resetting. Good fasting foods, the scientists describe, include fruit, light soups, salads, unbuttered toast, and half pieces of bread. Calories and carbohydrates should be kept to a minimum.

Summarized with the permission of the Argonne National Laboratory, Argonne, Illinois.

For a free, wallet-size copy of the diet, send a self-addressed, stamped envelope to Public Affairs, Argonne National Laboratory, 9700 South Cass Avenue, Argonne, IL 60439 (708/252-2000). For more information about the philosophy and research behind the diet, look in your local bookstore for *Overcoming Jet Lag* by Dr. Charles F. Ehret and Lynne Waller Scanlon (Berkeley Publications, 1987, 160 pages, $7.95).

Anxiety and Attitude

Stress produces some of the same symptoms as jet lag, and compounds others. If flight anxiety is an issue for you, you may be surprised to discover that once it's under control, a large part of what you thought was jet lag disappears.

The cause of jet lag is grounded in physical phenomena; it

is not a psychosomatic affliction. As is true elsewhere in life, however, the boundaries separating mind and body blur. When you fly, take a good attitude with you. Positive momentum will smooth the lines between time zones, giving your body extra energy for graceful adjustment.

Please don't try to follow all the advice in this book! At least not all at once. Don't let the attempt to become more comfortable turn into a burdensome list of must-do's and gizmos. We recommend that you hone in on those issues that are most important to you and concentrate on one at a time. On your next trip, work to stay hydrated. Carry that water bottle. The following trip, try the exercises, or one of the methods for minimizing jet lag. Go easy on yourself; no one can manage to incorporate too many new routines at once.

You'll probably find that not everything we mention strikes your fancy. Pick and choose. Our job was to cover the territory as thoroughly as possible, knowing that each person's comfort issues are unique. Your job is to decide how much effort you're willing to expend—changing habits or acquiring travel aids—based on your own tolerances, health philosophy, budget, and how far and often you fly. It's for you to decide whether the effects of dehydration warrant investing in a HumidiFlyer. It's for you to decide whether the ease of using new rolling luggage justifies its cost. NoiseBuster headphones are not for everyone.

We don't claim that air travel will be as enjoyable as stretching out on sun-dazzled sands or curling up in front of the fire on a snowy afternoon. But we do believe that most travelers' flying experiences can be significantly improved. We have included some tools for everyone and are confident you will find the ones you need.

So, good flights to you.

Appendix A:
Additional Information for Flyers

Flying with Children

"Whenever I hear a baby crying on the airplane," a woman traveling in business suit and heels declared, "I just want to stick my finger in its mouth."

If you're worried about her intentions, don't be. This woman knows the best way to help an infant adjust to air pressure changes: suckling. Why do infants and young children tend to cry during takeoff and landing? Their ears are plugged up and it hurts. By nursing, offering your baby a bottle or pacifier, or giving her your own finger to suckle, you can trigger an instinct that helps your infant unpop her ears.

The key to flying successfully with children is to anticipate their needs. It does take extra energy, but a little insight and preparation can transform your young ones into good traveling companions.

The annual airline issue of *Family Travel Times* is an unparalleled source of information about current issues concerning, and amenities available for, young flyers and their oft-frazzled parents. This special issue can be purchased for $12; a full subscription ($55) includes ten issues, discounts on other Travel with Your Children publications, and free trip consultation. *Family Travel Times*, c/o Travel with Your Children, 45 West 18th Street, 7th Floor Tower, New York, NY 10011 (212/206-0688).

Preboarding with children is a good idea. You can show your children the main features of the plane, take a peek in the cockpit, and get everyone tucked away and belted in before the crowd arrives.

Crying and Other Disturbances

When your baby cries, for whatever reason, take note of your own body language. Are you hunching over, worried about the noise and the disturbance? This may feel like disapproval to your child and certainly conveys tension. Try to relax. Let go of worry about what other passengers are thinking and be nurturing.

With older children, make a point to talk about flying before departure day. Tell them what to expect and answer questions about the trip. Use the car and paper experiments in Chapter Four to illustrate aerodynamics.

TIP There are a variety of entertaining and informative children's books about flying that can dispel anxiety and increase enjoyment of the trip. Take your child to your local bookstore or library and let him pick out his own.

Arrange gentle code words for "keep the noise down," "I need your attention," and other messages you or your child anticipate needing. Assigning code words ahead of time helps reduce stress in moments of conflict and empowers both parties—you and your child—with the responsibility for maintaining good communication.

The Price of the Ticket

Do children need tickets? The rules vary from airline to airline, so inquire when booking tickets. United Airlines, for example, allows *one* child under two years of age per accompanying adult to travel free on domestic flights, but that child has no checked baggage allowance. No seat can be reserved for children without tickets, so you may end up having to hold her in your lap; flying at unpopular hours is a good idea.

Even if the child has a reserved seat, a sparsely populated airplane gives the kids more room to spread out and will help you be less self-conscious about noise, restlessness, and frequent trips to the bathroom.

You may want to bring along an infant safety seat. Industry experts, including the FAA, agree this is the safest way for infants and toddlers to travel. You can use the same buckle-in chair you use for car travel if it's certified for use in an aircraft (if made in the mid-1980s or later, it should be okay) and will fit on a single seat.

For a free copy of the brochure, "Child/Infant Safety Seats Recommended for Use in Aircraft," call the FAA's Consumer Division (800/FAA-SURE or 202/267-3479).

If you've paid a child's fare for your baby, reserve a seat and plunk down your safety unit without asking. If you haven't bought a ticket for your child, make sure your safety seat can be stowed like any carry-on in case there's no empty seat available. Cabin personnel may be able to check the seat in the last minutes before flight, but don't count on it.

TIP If a reservations agent says you can use your safety seat without buying an extra ticket, request that the policy be noted in your computer passenger record. Call back a little later to make sure the notation is there. If any question arises at the gate, you're safe; airline personnel will defer to the details of your record.

Parents traveling without safety seats are asked to hold children under two in their laps, securing the belt around both of them during takeoffs, landings, and turbulence. Only one extra infant or small child is allowed per row (there are four oxygen masks available to every row of three seats). Some airlines offer extremely low infant fares that encourage parents to buy an extra ticket for children under two—securing a site for their seat. A few offer infant restraints, free of charge, to passengers.

Bassinets are provided free of charge on some domestic and many international aircraft. When making your reservations, you can request a seat assignment in an appropriate location for the bassinet—usually in the bulkhead row. Most bassinets are large enough to hold a child up to around six months old, but double-check by offering your child's size and weight. Take your own blanket to line the bottom. During takeoff, landing, or any time the fasten seatbelt sign is lit, parents must remove their children from bassinets and hold them in their laps.

Children aged two to eleven and accompanied by an adult may qualify for discounted tickets. Ask your travel agent to explore options from airline to airline.

What's Onboard, and What's Not

Ask your reservationist if there's a complimentary baby kit available on your flight. The contents may come in handy even though you bring your own supplies. A typical baby kit includes baby powder, a few disposable diapers, a bowl, a spoon, and baby food. While the flight attendants are happy to heat anything in hot water *when there's time,* airplanes are not equipped with bottles. You'd be well advised to board with all the (bottled) formula or milk you think you'll need.

TIP Parents who fly often recommend taking along several resealable plastic bags. They can be used for anything—food, toys, and supplies—and used again. They are particularly useful for the inevitable mess; seal and tuck them in a carry-on without worry. Try it. You'll wonder how you ever survived without them.

No matter how old your children are, take extra juice to stimulate swallowing, and keep them occupied during take-off and landing. Provide your children with something to eat; sucking and chewing will help their ears pop. Crackers work well, or anything that's crisp, clutchable, and not too sticky.

See who can eat their treat the most vigorously and make both ears pop before anyone else's. Give infants a bottle. Talk to kids about what happens during the popping (see Chapter Twelve), and make a game of it to keep their minds off the discomfort. Tell them they're training to climb Mt. Kilimanjaro.

TIP If your children are traveling with colds or are prone to earaches, consider these three aids: (1) A children's-strength decongestant, taken about an hour before takeoff and again before landing; (2) Vick's or eucalyptus oil to dot under noses and expand nasal passages; or (3) Ear Ease, a small, plastic-cup-like device that expands the Eustachian tubes and relieves pressure-related ear pain. (See Chapter Twelve.)

Finally, and perhaps most crucially, remember that children get dehydrated, too. They will find adequate liquid intake even more difficult to maintain than you do. Help your kids stay hydrated; pack plenty of water and juices.

Food and Games

You'll want to pack food for the rest of the flight, too. Even if you've ordered a kid's meal, it may not arrive when you need it. Kids have a harder time adjusting to new schedules than adults do. Don't count on getting supplies at the airport; you may only find ice cream, bruised apples, and overpriced pretzels from which to choose.

Take fun food from home: raisins; trail mix with nuts, other dried fruits, and chocolate; graham crackers; "ants on a log" (peanut butter spread thickly in the crease of celery sticks, with raisin "ants" walking along the top); boxed juices; and "fruit leather" dried-fruit rolls. Also appealing are sandwiches, gingerbread or ginger snaps (the ginger will help avert mild cases of motion sickness), and homemade, unsalted popcorn—don't worry, a cleaning crew will take care of any fallout.

TIP Some airlines serve meals to children first if asked. We recommend asking.

TIP Some airlines will present birthday cakes to kids for minimal or no cost. Ask, and order, when making reservations.

Most airlines offer some kind of activity kit for kids. This kit usually contains crayons, activity books, flight pins, and the like. We recommend packing one yourself. Include food and juice, a favorite toy that doesn't have lots of parts or require much space, and a familiar picture book. Get excited about reading it. Multiple times. The coup de grace will be a new surprise you smuggle into the kit when no one's looking. New, by definition, is enthralling for most children. Try a small, bendy toy for younger kids, origami paper with diagrams, silly putty, a new story cassette or book.

If you don't have time to pack your own, call S.W.A.K. (Sealed With A Kiss). Specify age and gender of your child; owner Julie Winston will custom pack a colorful, intriguing activity kit and send it along for about $30. Winston keeps a file on each customer so there's no repetition (800/888-SWAK or 301/468-2604).

Your child may also want to travel with a friend—a stuffed animal or special blanket. A portable tape player may be a good idea, along with audio cassettes, but help your kids pay attention to crew regulations about ascent and descent, when electronic devices must be turned off. Consider buying a copy of Marie Boatness's absolutely inspired book *Travel Games for the Family.*

Travel Games for the Family: 100 Ways to Entertain Kids of All Ages for Hours, by Marie Boatness (Canyon Creek Press, 1993, 133 pages, $9.95).

If your child is old enough, give him the responsibility for carrying his own bag, keeping track of it, and stowing everything neatly under the seat.

Layovers

Five hours in St. Louis—just you, six carry-ons, and the kids. What can you do?

▪ Secure your luggage and take everybody for an exploratory walk.

▪ Ask children to lead everyone—everyone in your travel group or, heck, everyone at the gate; no doubt they could use it—through stretches or a movement routine. You'd be surprised how much of the fitness movement is absorbed by kids. They know how to do it, and they know their bodies in a spontaneous, easy way many of us have forgotten. Play Simon Says. Don't be shy. Do the hoochie-koochie.

▪ Pull out the fun food snacks you've packed.

▪ Settle into a carpeted corner near your gate, make a fort with the luggage and play games. Again, we recommend Marie Boatness' *Travel Games* or another activity resource like it. Try the children's section at your local library for ideas. Bring cards; get a deck from a flight attendant or buy them at an airport store. Carry crayons (also available on many flights), borrow paper, and draw the planes. Draw other travelers walking by. Draw on postcards to send to a neighbor.

▪ If your kids know the alphabet, or can follow along with a little coaching, play a travel memory game incorporating objects around the airport. For example: "When I go flying, I take my apple." "When *I* go flying, I take my apple and my baggage." "Well, when *I* go flying, I take my apple, my baggage, my crayons, and…my detonator." Just kidding. Actually, joking about bombs or hijacking is *not* funny in an airport and can lead to arrest. Nor are children's plastic guns or knives appropriate for amusement during air travel. Weapon look-alikes are usually confiscated at security checks. Spare your children, airport officials, and yourself the trauma; take other toys.

TIP If you're flying Delta, ask about Dusty's Dens. Delta is opening a series of child amusement centers in airports, with games, snacks, and more.

KidsPort play areas can be found at a growing number of airports, including Pittsburgh International, Boston's Logan Airport, Denver International Airport, San Jose International (CA), Missoula International (MT), and LaGuardia (limited facilities). KidsPorts differ from one location to another but are free of charge, fun, educational play places geared to travelers between the ages of three and sixteen.

Children Flying Solo

Each U.S. airline has its own rules about unaccompanied children. Every parent has his own level of comfort with the thought—and so does his child! Here are a few guidelines that will help with the planning:

- In general, children under five are not allowed to travel without a responsible adult.

- Children between the ages of five and seven may fly by themselves on flights that require no change of plane (direct or nonstop).

- Between the ages of eight and eleven, children can travel unaccompanied but may be charged an additional fee. Notify the ticket agent when making reservations.

- Airlines may refuse to book unaccompanied children on afternoon or evening flights if they feel the child is at risk of missing connecting flights. They don't want to provide a chaperone to take care of the child if he's stranded overnight.

- If your child flies unaccompanied, you'll have to give the airline your name, phone number, and address; they'll need the same information about the adult scheduled to meet your child. Some airlines require a signature of release when the child is collected, and some require a photo ID.

- Young people aged twelve and above are considered adults by the airlines but can get help making connections. Again, ask when making reservations.

As a parent or guardian, it's up to you to determine whether or not your child is mature—and adventuresome—enough to travel alone. Pack drinks, snacks, and diversions for your child to take with her. Introduce her to the gate attendant, and tell the attendant that she is traveling alone. An airline attendant should take her under his wing before your child gets on the plane and will probably preboard with her so she can get situated. Make sure your child knows to wait, in her seat, for a flight attendant escort at the end of the flight.

Make sure the child is traveling with some spending money for movie headsets, or phone calls in case of delay. Prepare her by describing which services will be free—and which won't—during travel. Make sure she knows how to use a pay phone and make a collect call.

TIP Pack an itinerary and important emergency phone numbers in a pocket, or a pouch around her neck. Make sure to include the number of the person scheduled to meet her at the other end.

Talk to your child about interacting with strangers. You won't want to frighten her, but you may want to discuss appropriate versus inappropriate behavior, and what she can do if she feels uncomfortable (i.e., get up and go to a flight attendant or other adult).

TIP Consider choosing an aisle seat for your child. This affords more room for moving around and easier access to flight attendants.

Some airlines provide brochures for parents of children flying alone or for the children themselves. Ask when making reservations.

Pregnant Passengers

You are generally welcome to fly until you are eight months pregnant, after which time most airlines will refuse you at the gate. The concern here is airline liability, not passenger safety; sudden or extreme changes in pressure can induce labor. Check with the airline to ascertain their policy before making reservations.

It's also probably a good idea to discuss travel plans with your physician. If you are less than eight months pregnant but appear to be more, carry a dated note from your doctor in case questions arise. Feel free to preboard if you need the extra time to get settled. See Chapter Seven for chair and seatbelt suggestions.

Dramamine (and other antihistamines) and scopolamine ear patches are not recommended for pregnant or nursing women. The medication can be passed from mother to baby and may contribute to developmental defects. See Chapter Seventeen for safe alternatives.

Air Travelers with Disabilities

While progress toward a barrier-free environment for everyone who wants to fly is being made, the challenge of outdated facilities and general ignorance remains. Sight-impaired passengers are still met with wheelchairs. The president of the Paralyzed Veteran's Association of America is left sitting on the tarmac, his wheelchair flown to another city. Hearing-impaired passengers wait at the gate while loudspeakers broadcast their flight's delay—or cancellation.

Over forty-three million people in the United States with some form of disability need access to the sky for work- or pleasure-related travel. Airline passengers with disabilities routinely encounter inappropriate communication, a lack of understanding regarding their needs, and inadequate passenger and assistive-device transport. There are, however, a number of organizations working to improve conditions for the traveler with disabilities.

We urge everyone—not just the traveler with disabilities—to take part in this effort. In the meantime, the airline passenger with disabilities will have to plan well, understand the services guaranteed by law, and take appropriate action when his rights as an airline passenger have not been respected.

Access to the Skies, a program supported by the Paralyzed Veterans of America, publishes an extremely informative quarterly newsletter on air travel accessibility issues—and it's free! Access to the Skies also sponsors a semiannual accessibility conference. For information, or to get on the mailing list, contact Managing Editor Michelle Meacham, The Paralysis Society of America, ATTS Program, 801 18th Street N.W., Washington, DC 20006 (800/424-8200 ext. 790; TDD: 202/416-7622).

Your Rights as an Airline Passenger

The U.S. Air Carrier Access Act prohibits certain airline practices that passengers with disabilities have long considered inconsistent and arbitrary. As a result, the FAA, airlines, and airline personnel are now required to accommodate the needs of people with disabilities as they do the needs of all passengers—safely, quickly, and with dignity.

▪ Carriers may not refuse transportation to individuals on the basis of disability, nor may they limit the number of disabled persons on a flight.

▪ Carriers may not require advance notice that a disabled person is flying, but they may require up to forty-eight hours' notice for those accommodations that require preparation (transportation of an electric wheelchair on a small aircraft, providing hazardous-materials packaging for spillable batteries, accommodations for ten or more passengers with disabilities who travel as a group, etc.). Other services that may or may not be offered, including medical oxygen onboard, incubator carriage, and respirator hookup, also require twenty-four hours' notice and a reasonable, nondiscriminatory fee.

TIP When shopping around for your ticket, ask about the airline's special services for people with disabilities. Services may include Braille briefing procedures, open captions on videos, visual displays of information broadcast by loudspeakers at gate areas, and procedures for packaging battery-powered wheelchairs. When you book a ticket, ask for written confirmation, *including notation of any special service you have requested,* from the airline or travel agent.

▪ New and recently remodeled aircraft of a certain size must provide access facilities, including movable aisle armrests on half the aisles in the aircraft, accessible lavatories (with onboard chairs), and priority space for storing a personal wheelchair in the cabin.

▪ Carriers may not insist that anyone travel with an attendant, except in certain, very limited circumstances. If a traveler with disabilities and the carrier disagree about whether these circumstances exist, the carrier may require an attendant, but the carrier cannot charge for the transportation of the attendant.

▪ Carriers must provide boarding assistance, but they are not required to hand carry a passenger onboard a small plane when a lift or other boarding device is not an option.

TIP Tipping is not necessary or expected when airline personnel provide extra services, such as escort or carriage between connecting flights.

- Wheelchairs and other assistive devices have priority for in-cabin storage space, but only when these aids make it on-board first; no assistive device can displace the carry-on items already stowed by other passengers.

- Other provisions of the act concern the treatment of mobility aids and assistive devices (including the dismantling of personally owned wheelchairs and the packaging of spillable batteries), access to routine passenger information, accommodations for persons with hearing impairments, security screening, communicable diseases and medical certificates, and service animals.

TIP Talking boards and the like (augmentative and alternative communication devices) do not threaten the safe operation of aircraft. When the pilot commands that all electronic devices be shut off below a certain altitude, he's not talking about these, which emit no interfering signal, or radio wave. He is talking about laptop computers and video games, which do.

- Carriers must have established systems for fielding complaints, including on-the-spot "complaints resolution officials" and procedures for responding to written criticisms. Any passenger who believes she has been unfairly treated should file her grievance with the airline and with the DOT's Office of Consumer Affairs, 400 Seventh Street S.W., Washington, DC 20590.

A pamphlet with detailed explanation of all rights guaranteed to the passenger with a disability, *New Horizons for the Air Traveler with a Disability,* can be obtained free of charge by contacting the DOT (202/366-2220; TDD: 202/755-7687).

These regulations do not apply to non-U.S. airlines, or airport facilities outside the U.S., but do apply to international transportation by U.S. carriers. Travelers should be aware that the facilities that exist in the U.S. may not be available abroad; most travel agents can provide information about the conditions and requirements for traveling abroad as a disabled passenger.

Mobility International, USA, is a national nonprofit organization whose purpose is to promote and facilitate international educational exchange and travel opportunities for people with disabilities. Information sheets about the accessibility of many overseas destinations are available to members (individual membership is $20 per year). Other benefits include a quarterly newsletter and discounts on select publications. For more information, contact: Mobility International, USA, P.O. Box 10767, Eugene, OR 97440; (V/TDD: 503/343-1284; fax: 503/343-6812; E-mail: miusa@igc.apc.org).

The Society for Advancement of Travel for the Handicapped (SATH) publishes resource sheets with accessibility information, particularly for international travel. Annual membership varies: $25 for seniors and students, $45 for individuals, and $100 for travel agencies. For more information, contact Peter Shaw-Lawrence, Executive Director, SATH, 347 Fifth Avenue, Suite 610, New York, NY 10016 (212/447-SATH).

Paving the Way for a Smooth Flight

Careful planning is the key here.

- Ask your travel or ticket agent all the necessary questions to make sure you're scheduled to fly on a plane that offers the facilities you need.

- Plan ahead for travel with a companion when necessary.

- Book early to reserve seats that offer the most comfort and convenience.

- Allow plenty of extra time before and between flights—for security checks, transport to and from the gates, preboarding, and individual safety briefing where necessary.

- Place a request in advance if you want a wheelchair from the ticket counter to the gate, between flights, or from final deplaning to the baggage claim area. You may want to confirm your request the day before flying.

- Call your destination airport or airports to find out about terminal accessibility. Local TDD numbers are often listed in the phone book; either local information or your travel agent can help you if they're not. Most people don't notice the things they don't need, so direct questions work best. Rather than posing a blanket question about available facilities, go down the list of specifics.

Inquire about accessible parking areas near the terminal and appropriate signs and guides to find them; accessible medical and traveler's aid stations; accessible restrooms and drinking fountains; accessible ticketing systems; amplified and text (TDD) telephones, visual and verbal paging systems; accessible baggage check-in and retrieval areas; accessible jetways and mobile lounges; level entry boarding ramps, lifts or other means of assisting an individual with a disability on and off an aircraft; directional signs indicating the locations of these facilities and services; and anything else you need.

Access Travel: Airports, a comprehensive guide to the accessibility of terminals worldwide, is produced by Airports Council International. Access Travel: Airports includes useful medical traveling tips, information about the Air Carrier Access and Americans with Disabilities acts, and a solid listing of toll-free voice and TDD numbers for airlines, rental car agencies, and international hotel chains. Single, free copies can be obtained by sending a written request to Consumer Information Center, Pueblo, CO 81009.

Traveling with Animals

Airlines require crates for traveling animals. These can be purchased in different sizes from most Humane Society Shelters, pet stores, your local vet's office—even some airlines.

For dogs, cats, and domesticated birds weighing twenty pounds or less, carry-on is an option. Make a reservation for your pet when you book your tickets, or as soon as possible thereafter; on most aircraft, only two carry-on animals are allowed in coach, one in first class. There is an additional charge for flying with your pet, usually around $50.

Your pet must fit under the seat in front of you (no animals overhead), and travel in a small, hard-sided kennel or a soft-sided pet carrier. While the soft carriers fit most readily under the seat, a spokesperson from the Humane Society describes fiberglass or plastic hard-sided kennels as "easier on the animal" because the floor and sides won't cave or crush.

Nine airlines have given their approval to the Sherpa Bag pet carrier, with front and top zippers, easy-to-clean bottom, and sturdy mesh on the sides for ventilation and a good view. The bag's adjustable shoulder strap comes off as a leash. The whole thing looks like a padded sports bag, and fits easily under the seat; approximately $60 to $70, depending on size. See Appendix B for mail-order sources.

A passenger pet enjoys almost as many rights as its owner. If any human passenger is allergic to your pet, it's not your responsibility; that passenger will have to try to change seats or take a later flight.

Many pet owners worry about sending their best friends as

"checked luggage," but it's really not so traumatic. Unfamiliar and perhaps uncomfortable, but serving a greater purpose. Your animal will be placed, snug in his kennel, in the belly of the plane. You'd be surprised at the number of compassionate souls working in baggage who will ease your friend's trip with low, comforting voices and a little extra attention. If you're worried, you may want to discuss with your vet the pros and cons of using tranquilizers.

The charge for sending your pets by air is higher when you're not onboard. The transcontinental price for a twenty-five-pound unaccompanied animal is usually around $100; final price is determined by weight but differs from airline to airline. The best mode of travel for pets going solo is an airline's priority shipping service, not regular cargo. Priority shipping guarantees animals the least time in transit. Priority animals are the last to go aboard, the first to leave, and are scheduled to make tight connections instead of the three and a half hours required for cargo. Shipped animals can usually be picked up at the airline's baggage office in the airport's baggage service area.

American Airlines boasts the best record for shipping live animals, and their stringent health and climactic stipulations illustrate why. American's guidelines are as follows:

▪ The animal must arrive at the airport with two copies of a health certificate, both dated within ten days of travel, as well as a rabies vaccination certificate less than one year old.

▪ The temperature of origin, connecting, and destination cities must be between 45° and 85° Fahrenheit. Reservations are taken one day in advance, using the forecasted highs for each area to make sure temperatures will be safe for animals.

▪ As the animal owner/shipper, American requires that you certify in writing that you offered the animal food and water within four hours of scheduled departure. When you arrive at the airport, the agent checking your pet will ask that you sign a statement to this effect. The document will then be affixed to the side of your animal's kennel.

▪ Animals must be shipped in kennels with separate compartments for food and water, both of which must be renewable without opening the kennel door. In the case of long flights or delays, baggage attendants will provide water for animals through kennel doors. If you tape a small bag of dry food and a list of instructions to the cage, attendants will feed your animal. If your animal is not to be fed, you must attach a note from your vet to that effect to the outside of the kennel.

Appendix B: Sources for Flight Books and Accessories

Travel bookstores and general bookstores with good travel sections are the best places to look for the books we recommend. If you don't have convenient access to either, there are excellent mail-order sources for travel books. The following put out mail-order catalogs:

Book Passage Bookstore
51 Tamal Vista Boulevard
Corte Madera, CA 94925
800/321-9785 or 415/924-3838

Christine Columbus
P.O. Box 2137
Lake Oswego, OR 97035-0643
800/280-4775 or 503/697 0968; fax: 800/803-5383

Globe Corner Bookstore
One School Street
Boston, MA 02108
800/358-6013 or 617/523-6658

The Literate Traveler
8306 Wilshire Blvd., Suite 591
Beverly Hills, CA 90211
310/398-8781

Transit Books, Inc.
15 Mercer Road
Natick, MA 01760
800/998-0245

Travel accessories are available through a variety of sources. You may be able to find them in your area in travel bookstores, luggage stores, or specialty travel stores. There are also mail-order sources that offer a broad range of travel items. Gather catalogs and comparison shop from home.

Austin House

Previously a wholesale operation, Austin House is now offering inventory for direct sale via mail order. Offering more than a hundred travel-tested items and a catalog peppered with elucidating travel wisdom (a full page on the difference between the electricity adapters, converters, and transformers used for travel overseas, for example), Austin House offers a seventy-two-hour delivery guarantee. For a catalog, contact Austin House: P.O. Box 117, Station B, Buffalo, NY 14207 (800/268-5157 or 905/825-2650; fax: 800/469-5222 or 905/825-3200). Both toll-free numbers are good for use in the U.S. and Canada.

Brookstone

Slipped in among the arguably excessive tools and "time-savers" of the Brookstone catalog are a few slick, useful items aimed at the executive air traveler. The good news is, you don't have to be an executive to use them—or to afford them. For a catalog or local store listing, contact Brookstone at 17 Riverside Street, Nashua, NH 03062 (800/926-7000 or 314/581-7777; fax: 314/581-736).

Christine Columbus

A mail-order catalog that specializes in women's travel merchandise to make travel easier, safer, and more secure. Christine Columbus carries luggage, books (over sixty titles), clothing, footwear, and a wide array of travel accessories. Categories include: Traveling with Kids, Traveling Alone, Business and Leisure. To request a catalog, contact Christine Columbus at P.O. Box 2137, Lake Oswego, OR 97035-0643 (800/280-4775 or 503/697 0968; fax: 800/803-5383).

Eagle Creek Outfitters

Longtime producers of high-quality cordura nylon and canvas gear, Eagle Creek Outfitters emphasizes responsible travel. Their travel gear is designed to be functional, durable, comfortable, and convenient. By all reports, it is. The breadth of their duffle, backpack, pocket, and pouch offerings includes something for almost everyone—and everything is guaranteed for life. Eagle Creek also publishes a practical— though promotional—*Travel Gear Guide: A "How To" Guide on Travel Outfitting,* which they'll send you, free. Contact Eagle Creek for a *Guide,* or for the nearest Eagle Creek retailer: 1740 La Costa Meadows Drive, San Marcos, CA 92069 (800/874-9925 or 619/471-7600).

Magellan's Essentials for the Traveler

This catalog is issued once a year, the items handpicked and tested by owner John McManus and his staff. Customer service personnel are extremely knowledgeable. Every item is 100 percent guaranteed. For a catalog, contact Magellan's, Box 5485, Santa Barbara, CA 93150-5485 (800/962-4943 or 805/568-5400; fax: 805/568-5406).

Appendix C:
Consumer Flying Publications

Condé Nast Traveler
This glamorous-looking monthly magazine almost always contains one full-length article and numerous tidbits on flying. Recent exposés include a low-down on cabin air, thorough discussion of melatonin therapy, and financial evaluation of first-class and business services. Well written and, frankly, entertaining. Annual subscription rate is $15, per-issue newsstand price is $3.95. For more information, contact *Condé Nast Traveler*, 350 Madison Avenue, New York, NY 10017 (800/777-0700 or 303/666-7000).

Consumer Reports Travel Letter
A thorough and aggressive newsletter, especially where discount fares, economical car rental, and frequent flyer mileage accrual are concerned. Ed Perkins, editor, is a discerning and fearless reviewer. The average issue is twenty-four pages and is published twelve times each year. Annual subscription rate: $39.00. For more information, contact: *Consumer Reports Travel Letter*, P.O. Box 53629, Boulder, CO 80322 (800/234-1645 or 303/666-7000).

Consumer Reports Travel Buying Guide
This annual publication is the product of Ed Perkins and the other editors at *Consumer Reports Travel Letter*. It covers a wide range of travel topics, including good airfare buys, charters, and consolidators. Consumer Reports Books, $8.99. Available in bookstores and through *Consumer Reports* (800/272-0722 or 515/237-4902).

Inside Flyer
Specifically geared to the mega-mileage flyer, *Inside Flyer* goes to great lengths to educate readers about specific frequent flyer options and bargains. The typical issue is thirty-six pages and is published twelve times a year. Annual

subscription rate is $33 For more information, contact *Inside Flyer*, 4715-C Town Center Drive, Colorado Springs, CO 80916 (719/597-8889).

Index

Access to the Skies, 171. *See also* disability, travelers with

Access Travel: Airports (Airports Council International), 175. *See also* disability, travelers with

aerodontalgia, 107

aerodynamic principles of control, lift, and thrust, 47–48, 50

aerophobia: definition and common causes of, 19–20; fear and control, 17–18; fearful flyer programs and therapy for, 63. *See also* guided imagery; desensitization

affirmations. *See* positive messages

Air Carrier Access Act, 171–73. *See also* disability, travelers with

airlines, commercial: on time arrival performance of, 68; luggage handling ratings for, 90; fearful flyer programs, 63; meal preparation, 81–83. *See also* contract, airline; luggage

air pressure changes and effects on body, 103–4, 106–7

air quality. *See* ventilation, airplane

air traffic, affects of heavy, 67

air traffic control, 57–58

alcohol consumption: and dehydration, 111; and jet lag, 155; and motion sickness, 130

anchor points: and day of flight, 46; technique for establishing, 38–45. *See also* guided imagery

animals. *See* pets

anxiety. *See* aerophobia

baby kit, 165–66. *See also* children

baggage. *See* luggage

beta blockers, 132–33. *See also* motion sickness

boarding, 99

boarding pass, 79–80

breathing for posture and relaxation, 116–18. *See also* guided imagery; ventilation, airplane

bulkhead row, seating in, 74, 76

bumping regulations, strategies, and compensation, 144–46

business class. *See* seat selection

cabin baggage, 91

cable lock, retractable, 147–48

calling cards, 149

cancellations, flight, 143–44

carry-on luggage, 90–92. *See also* pets

chapel, airport, 149

check-in, advantages to early, 98–99

children: and ear pain, 163, 166; entertainment for, 167–69; safety seats and seat selection for, 78, 164–65; sitting near, 136–37; snacks and meals for, 83, 86,

166–67; ticketing requirements for, 164–65; on unaccompanied flights, 169–70

circulation, 120–21

clear air turbulence, 53

clubs, airport, 149–50

coach. *See* seat selection

cockpit, visiting, 99

compensation. *See* contract, airline

computer equipment: club facilities for, 149–50; and security checkpoints, 102

conditions of carriage. *See* contract, airline

confirmation, flight, 68, 80

connecting flight, 69

contract, airline: concerning delays, cancellations, and overbooking, 142–46; filing complaint upon breach of, 141; negotiating, 142, 146;

control, aerodynamic principle of, 50

cruising altitude and speed, 55

dehydration, 108, 111–13

de-icing airplane, 52

delays, flight, 142–43

dental work, flight restrictions due to, 107

Department of Transportation. *See* DOT

desensitization, techniques for, 62–63

Diet, The Anti-Jet Lag, 157–59

digestion and air pressure changes, 106

direct flight, 69

disability, travelers with: Access to the Skies, 171; *Access Travel: Airports*, 175; Air Carrier Access Act, 171–73; DOT pamphlet for, 173; Mobility International USA, 173–74; preflight planning, 174–75; SATH, 174; seat selection, 77;

dispatchers, responsibilities of, 54–55

dizziness. *See* motion sickness

DOT (Department of Transportation): airline contract requirements under, 141, 144–146; filing a claim with, 96; *New Horizons for the Air Traveler with a Disability* pamphlet, 173

dramamine, 131. *See also* motion sickness

Ear Ease, 106

ear pain: causes of and remedies for, 103–4, 106; and children, 163, 166

ear patches, 132. *See also* motion sickness

excess valuation coverage, 97

exit row, seating in, 76

FAA (Federal Aviation Administration): air traffic control, 57–58; *Child/Infant Safety Seats Recommended for Use in Aircraft* brochure, 164; consumer safety hotline, 140; requirements for disabled travelers, 171–73; dispatchers, 54–55; inspection, 55–56; public education, 58; responsibilities of, 53–54

Facts & Advice for Airline Passengers (Aviation Consumer Action Project), 142

fantasy scenarios: body massage, 36; country meadow, 33; nurturing person, 34; a safe place, 35; white light, 37. *See also* guided imagery

Fearful Flyer's Resource Guide, The (Elkus and Tieger), 63

Federal Aviation Administration. *See* FAA

film and security checkpoints, 102
first class. *See* seat selection
flight attendants, training, 54
food. *See* meals
From Takeoff to Landing: Everything You Wanted to Know About Airplanes but Had No One to Ask (Gold and Sternstein), 50

ginger, 131. *See also* motion sickness
guided imagery, 21–22; active (progressive body) relaxation technique, 31–32; establishing anchor points, 38–45, 46; fantasy scenarios, 32–37; internal alarm clock, 23; positive messages, 30; relaxation technique, 22–29

hot cup method, 104, 106
HumidiFlyer mask, 113
hypnosis, 21–22. *See also* guided imagery

inspection. *See* FAA
insurance for luggage, 97
internal alarm clock, 23. *See also* guided imagery
isometric exercises, 120–21

jet lag: adjustment tips, 155–56; The Anti-Jet Lag Diet, 157–59; anxiety and, 159–60; melatonin to reduce, 156–57; symptoms and causes of, 154–55

KidsPort, 169. *See also* children

layover: with children, 168–69; creative uses for, 147–50, 152–53; scheduling a, 69–70
lift: aerodynamic principle of, 47–48; ascent and descent, 60, 61

lightning, 52
luggage: airline liability for damaged, late, or lost, 88, 89, 91, 94–97; carriers, 93–94; cart rental, 148; carry-on, 90–92; checking, 87–90; personal insurance for, 97; Travelpro Rollaboard, 92–93. *See also* pets

meals: availability of special, 82–83; brown bag, 83–84, 86; preparation of, 81–82. *See also* Diet, The Anti-Jet Lag
melatonin, 156–57. *See also* jet lag
Mobility International USA, 173–74. *See also* disability, travelers with
motion sickness: causes and symptoms of, 128–29, 133; preventative tips and medication for, 129–33

nausea. *See* motion sickness
neck pillow, 124, 126
New Horizons for the Air Traveler with a Disability (DOT), 173. *See also* disability, travelers with
noise control, 122–23, 137
nonsmoking seating on domestic and international flights, 76–77, 113–14
nonstop flight, 69

OAG (Official Airline Guides): *Pocket Flight Guide*, 69; *Travel Planner*, 152
office center, airport, 153
overbooking. *See* bumping
Overcoming Jet Lag (Ehret and Scanlon), 159

pets: avoiding carry-on, 78; traveling with, 175–77, 91
pilot: communication from, 60–61;

plane inspection by, 56; training, 54

Pocket Flight Guide (OAG), 69

positive messages, 30. *See also* guided imagery

posture: and breathing, 116–18; upper body and lower back adjustment, 117–121

pregnancy: restrictions, 170–71; seat selection, 77

refund. *See* contract, airline

regulation. *See* FAA

relaxation techniques. *See* guided imagery; posture

Rollaboard, Travelpro, 92–93

safety, airplane: consumer safety hotline, 140; international travel advisory information, 140; precautionary guidelines, 138–39; statistics on, 19

Salk's International Airport Transit Guide, 150

SATH (The Society for Advancement of Travel for the Handicapped), 174. *See also* disability, travelers with

scuba diving and flight restrictions, 107

seatbelt, 77

seat selection: changing, 78; class, dimension, and location specifications for, 71–74, 76; and particular objectives, 74, 76–78

security checkpoints, 100–1; carrying film and computers through, 102

self-hypnosis. *See* guided imagery

Shoulder Strap, Ultimate, 92

smoking, allowances and restrictions for, 76–77, 113–14

sounds, inflight, 58, 60–61

stretching, 120–21

temperature, airplane, 114–15

thrust, aerodynamic principle of, 48, 50

time zones, crossing, 68. *See also* jet lag

travel agent, 68, 69

Travel Planner (OAG), 152

turbulence: in descent and landing, 61; and weather, 51–53

Valsalva maneuver, 104

ventilation, airplane, 108–110. *See also* dehydration

weather, 51–53

wheelchair accessibility. *See* disability, travelers with

wind shears, 52

wing flaps, 50, 60, 61

wing flex, 50

wristbands, 132. *See also* motion sickness

Eighth Mountain books can be found in independent and chain bookstores across the U.S. and Canada. Books can also be ordered directly from the press. Please add $2.50 for the first book and 50¢ each additional book for postage and handling. Send a check (payable to The Eighth Mountain Press) to: 624 SE 29th Avenue, Portland, OR 97214. Books will be mailed book rate. If you need speedier delivery, call 503/233-3936 to discuss other options.

Eighth Mountain titles are distributed to the trade by Consortium Book Sales and Distribution, 1045 Westgate Drive, Saint Paul, MN 55114-1065 (800/283-3572 or 612/221-9035) and are carried by all major book wholesalers and library jobbers. For specialty and catalog sales contact Eighth Mountain directly at 624 SE 29th Avenue, Portland, OR 97214 (503/233-3936).

A Journey of One's Own
Uncommon Advice for the Independent Woman Traveler

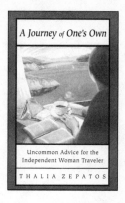

◆ Covers dozens of topics, including: dealing with sexual harassment, staying healthy, traveling safely, avoiding theft, and managing a trip of extended duration.

◆ "Superlatives generally make us suspicious, but we must say: **This is THE best women's travel resource we've seen, ever**.... It's authoritative; it's supportive; it's amusing; it really does have it all."—*New York Daily News*

$14.95
360 pages
trade paperback
ISBN 0-933377-36-3

◆ "Zepatos is teacher, spokeswoman and heroine of sorts to a generation of travelers, both women and men, who understand travel as more than the periodic recreational migration that our commercial culture promotes."—*Seattle Times*

OTHER TRAVEL BOOKS FROM THE EIGHTH MOUNTAIN PRESS

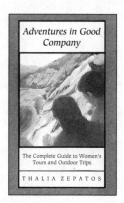

$16.95
432 pages
trade paperback
ISBN 0-933377-27-4

Adventures in Good Company
The Complete Guide to Women's Tours and Outdoor Trips

◆ Profiles over 100 companies worldwide.

◆ Covers the whole range of outdoor excursions—bicycling, canoeing, kayaking, rock climbing, horseback riding, sailing, dog sledding, trekking, etc.—as well as international tours, spiritual journeys, and leadership development courses.

◆ Explores issues particular to group travel: how to choose a company and a trip, what your guide will expect of you and what you can expect of your guide, getting in shape, and how to organize your own group.

◆ "Warm, wise and wonderfully instructive...a beguiling blend of anecdotes, advice, and practical information."—*San Francisco Examiner and Chronicle*